I0647739

OTHER BOOKS IN THE YOGA MINIBOOK SERIES

*The Yoga Minibook for Energy and Strength*
*The Yoga Minibook for Longevity*
*The Yoga Minibook for Stress Relief*

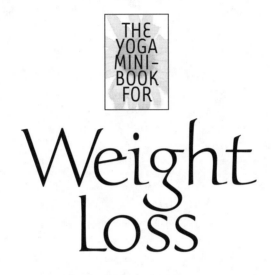

# THE YOGA MINI-BOOK FOR

# Weight Loss

A Specialized Program for a Thinner, Leaner You

## ELAINE GAVALAS

Illustrations by Nelle Davis

A Fireside Book · Published by Simon & Schuster · New York London Toronto Sydney Singapore

FIRESIDE
Rockefeller Center
1230 Avenue of the Americas
New York, NY 10020

Copyright © 2003 by Elaine Gavalas

Illustrations copyright © 2003 by Nelle Davis

All rights reserved, including the right of reproduction
in whole or in part in any form.

FIRESIDE and colophon are registered trademarks of Simon & Schuster, Inc.

For information regarding special discounts for bulk purchases,
please contact Simon & Schuster Special Sales at 1-800-456-6798
or business@simonandschuster.com

Designed by Chris Welch

Manufactured in the United States of America

1    3    5    7    9    10    8    6    4    2

Library of Congress Cataloging-in-Publication Data
Gavalas, Elaine.
The yoga minibook for weight loss : a specialized program for a thinner, leaner
you/Elaine Gavalas.
p.    cm.
Includes index.
1.  Yoga—Health aspects.    2.  Weight loss.    I.  Title.
RA781.7. G378        2003
613.7'046—dc21                                                    2002026787
ISBN 0-7432-2698-4

DISCLAIMER

This publication contains the opinions and ideas of its author. It is intended to provide helpful and informative material on the subjects addressed in the publication. It is sold with the understanding that the author and publisher are not engaged in rendering medical, health, or any other kind of professional services in the book. The reader should consult his or her medical, health or other competent professional before adopting any of the suggestions in this book or drawing inferences from it.

The author and publisher specifically disclaim all responsiblity for any liability, loss, or risk, personal or otherwise, that is incurred as a consequence, directly or indirectly, of the use and application of any of the contents of this book.

For my guru, Katzy,
whose love and wisdom are the signposts on my path

# Acknowledgments

This book would not have been possible without the help and creative contributions of my husband and writing guru, Stuart Katz. His brilliant literary judgment and patient work helped me bring this text to life. I am forever grateful for his extraordinary love, friendship, and support.

I wish to offer my heartfelt thanks to all of the talented professionals at Simon & Schuster Trade Paperbacks for producing my yoga minibook series, with special thanks to Trish Todd for providing me with the opportunity to write the books, and to my editor, Lisa Considine, for her expertise and sage guidance.

I also wish to extend my deepest gratitude and appreciation to my literary agent, Michael Psaltis (and the Ethan Ellenberg Literary

Agency), for his wise counsel, encouragement, and support of my yoga books from the beginning.

I especially wish to thank Nelle Davis, who brought the yoga poses alive with her wonderful illustrations.

I am truly grateful to my parents-in-law, Ethel Katz Regolini and Leo Regolini, and my uncles, Arthur Vozeolas and Henry Kane, for their wisdom, help, and guidance.

Finally, many thanks to my yoga teachers (with special gratitude to Ram Dass), and to you, dear reader. May yoga bring you lasting health, happiness, peace, longevity, freedom, and bliss. *Om shanthi* with love.

# Contents

# chapter 1

# Understanding Yoga

Are you one of the millions of people trying to lose weight, or trying not to gain it all back? Weight control is a common problem, so if you answered yes, you're certainly not alone. Over the years, I've worked with many people just like you, who have similar questions and concerns, such as the following: With the proliferation of fitness trends, how do you choose the best weight management plan for your body's needs? When you've had enough of trendy programs, how can you maintain your weight loss?

You hold the answers to these questions in your hands. I've written *The Yoga Minibook for Weight Loss* for everyone who is tired of being disappointed, let down, fed up, exhausted, and dizzy from riding the unhealthy dietary-fad roller coaster. The yoga program described in this book approaches weight management in a unique way that will integrate your body, mind, and spirit. By following this program you can safely and successfully lose pounds and inches. You can also redistribute your weight while firming and toning your out-of-shape areas. Best of all, the gentle stretching, strengthening, and firming poses in the pages that follow are suitable for people at all levels of fitness and flexibility. Yoga for Weight Loss is a lifestyle program that will help you achieve and maintain your desired weight goals, make the best fitness and food choices, and enrich your mind.

Exercise fads come and go, but after more than five thousand years, the practice of yoga is still with us—and more popular than ever. Most weight loss plans ultimately prove to be fads, offering short-term solutions to a long-term problem. Most people find these plans impossible to stay on for a prolonged period of time. In contrast, the Yoga for Weight Loss program is based on a fundamentally sound, totally different approach. The practice of yoga offers a positive change in lifestyle, where permanent weight loss is a natural by-product of enjoyable exercise.

At the core of the program is a routine that features *vinyasa* yoga practice, a series of postures that flow seamlessly from one to the next. It's a dynamic combination of yoga and aerobics that will help you burn calories, raise your metabolism, and promote your cardiovascular health. With my Yoga Power workout you'll melt off pounds, increase your strength and flexibility, and stretch your spiritual muscles all at once.

If excess weight around your stomach is your nemesis, try practicing yoga poses from the "Yoga for Abdominals" chapter. Just a few minutes a day will help you create and maintain that sleek, sensual stomach you've always dreamed about. If you're concerned about unsightly cellulite or flabby, out-of-shape muscles, the "Yoga for Toning" chapter can get you firm, lean, and fit with supersculpting yoga postures. This yoga workout has the power to transform your body. It will tone you from head to toe, help you lose fat, encourage good posture, build muscle, and reduce the appearance of cellulite.

Yoga is not just for skinny, ultraflexible, beautiful people, although the media often portray it that way. On the contrary, the greatest boon is that yoga most benefits those who need it the most. The "Gentle Yoga" chapter is for beginners and people with full-sized bodies, who may be intimidated by the challenge of more advanced, pretzel-like yoga poses. Although some yoga postures may look difficult, remember that yoga is noncompetitive and emphasizes self-acceptance. With patient and regular practice you can safely and gradually increase your workout intensity and fitness level, regardless of your size or shape.

For valuable information on yoga nutrition and eating, the "Yoga Food" chapter includes a sampling of the world's healthiest cuisines—the Mediterranean, vegetarian, Asian, and ayurvedic diets. By incorporating the yoga principles of Ayurveda and the foods of these deliciously healthful cuisines into your eating style, you'll give yourself an opportunity to achieve and maintain your perfect weight and feel your very best. In that chapter you'll also find helpful ways to modify your eating habits, such as practicing mindful eating and scaling down your food portions yet still feeling satisfied.

*The Yoga Minibook for Weight Loss* also features tips on how to incorporate yoga into your everyday life, along with ways to develop your personal yoga practice. I've created Yoga for Weight Loss to help people of all sizes, shapes, and ages reach and maintain their ideal weight and fitness goals, through sustained individualized practice and good lifelong eating habits.

Over the years, I have studied and practiced many hatha yoga styles, such as Integral, Iyengar, ashtanga vinyasa, kundalini, mantra, raja, and tantra, and have been especially interested in yoga's therapeutic applications. I have observed individuals and groups practicing yoga, and have seen its power to help them lose weight and relieve stress while they increase their energy, strength, and longevity. I've written my yoga minibook series—the first four being *The Yoga Minibook for Weight Loss, The Yoga Minibook for Longevity, The Yoga Minibook for Stress Relief,* and *The Yoga Minibook for Energy and Strength*—as self-help guides, in response to people's many fitness, diet, and wellness problems, questions, and concerns. I've had an opportunity to apply yoga techniques to help people achieve their wellness goals, and I've seen spectacular results.

My greatest wish is to share with you the many wonderful benefits yoga practice has given to me and the individuals I've assisted over the years. Whether you're looking to lose weight, boost your energy, relieve stress, or find the fountain of youth, I've created a yoga book for you. But before we dive in, a little background.

## 21st Century Yoga

Throughout the centuries, yoga has redefined and re-created itself to meet the needs of different eras and cultures. Yoga was barely known in the Western world until the 1960s, when the Beatles went off to India to find spiritual enlightenment with Maharishi Mahesh Yogi, and George Harrison came back with a sitar. Since then, yoga has evolved from a practice for hippie spiritual seekers chanting Om with Swami Satchidananda at Woodstock in 1969 to a practice embraced by everyone from Hollywood stars striving for beautiful bodies and high-powered CEOs seeking stress relief, to baby boomers wanting to turn back the hands of time. Even United States Supreme Court Justice Sandra Day O'Connor takes a weekly yoga class. At least fifteen million Americans include some form of yoga in their fitness regimen.

Although yoga has been celebrated as the new fitness philosophy for the twenty-first century, the practice of yoga actually goes back thousands of years. Yoga originated in India and is an ancient philosophical discipline, not a religion. Originally yoga was practiced as a path to spiritual enlightenment, a way of arriving at a state of pure bliss and oneness with the universe. *Yoga* is a Sanskrit word meaning "union"; it describes the integration of body, mind, and spirit, and communion with a universal energy, the Supreme Consciousness. The practice of hatha yoga, whose exercises are familiar to many Westerners, was originally devised to strengthen the body and prepare it for the long, motionless hours of meditation.

Yoga dates back to the ancient Vedas, sacred Hindu scriptures first recorded around 2500 B.C.E. Over millennia, the yoga tradition has evolved into eight principal branches, which are different paths that all lead to the same goal: enlightenment.

The eight branches of yoga are called the Wheel of Yoga. They are

**Hatha Yoga** (pronounced *haht-ha*), the yoga of physical discipline and bodily mastery. This is the branch of yoga most of us in the West are familiar with, and it is the one presented in this book. In hatha, enlightenment is achieved through spiritualized physical practices including *asana*s (postures), *pranayama* (controlled breathing), and meditation. The *Hatha Yoga Pradipika*, a fourteenth-century text, is a guide to hatha yoga.

**Jhana Yoga** (pronounced *gyah-nah*), the yoga of wisdom and knowledge. In jhana, enlightenment and self-realization are achieved through the teaching of nondualism, the elimination of illusion, and direct knowledge of the divine.

**Bhakti Yoga** (pronounced *bhuk-tee*), the path to achieve union with the divine through love and acts of devotion.

**Karma Yoga** (pronounced *kahr-mah*), the path of enlightenment through selfless service and actions.

**Mantra Yoga** (pronounced *mahn-trah*), the yoga of sacred sounds for self-awakening. A form of mantra yoga familiar to Westerners is Transcendental Meditation.

**Kundalini Yoga** (pronounced *koon-da-leenee*), the activation of the latent spiritual energy stored in the body and raised along the spine to the head through the breath and movement.

**Tantra Yoga** (pronounced *tahn-trah*), union with all that you are, achieved by harnessing sexual energy. Although tantra yoga has become famous for some rituals that spiritualize sexuality, it is essentially a spiritual discipline of nonsexual rituals and visualizations that activate spiritual energy.

**Raja Yoga** (pronounced *rah-jah*)—also known as royal, classical, eight-limbed, or *ashtanga* (not to be confused with the separate ashtanga style of yoga)—yoga of the mind and mental mastery. In the second century B.C.E., the great Hindu sage Patanjali wrote down the principles of classical yoga in the *Yoga Sutras*. Patanjali describes eight steps or "limbs" known as the Tree of Yoga. These eight limbs provide ethical guidelines for living and help along the yoga path to enlightenment.

The Tree of Yoga is composed of

**Yama** (pronounced *yah-mah*), the roots of the tree, which are moral discipline and ethical restraints. These include nonviolence *(ahimsa)*, truthfulness, freedom from avarice, chastity, and noncovetousness.

**Niyama** (pronounced *nee-yah-mah*), the trunk of the tree, which represents self-restraint and observance, including cleanliness, contentment, self-discipline, introspection or self-study, and devotion.

**Asana** (pronounced *ah-sah-nah*), the branches of the tree. It includes the postures of hatha yoga.

**Pranayama** (pronounced *prah-nah-yah-mah*), the leaves of the tree. It includes breath control for circulation of *prana*, or life-force energy.

**Pratyahara** (pronounced *prah-tyah-hah-rah*), the bark of the tree. It includes withdrawal of the senses for meditation.

**Dharana** (pronounced *dah-rah-nah*), the sap. It includes concentration for meditation.

**Dhyana** (pronounced *dee-yah-nah*), the flower. It includes meditation.

**Samadhi** (pronounced *sah-mah-dhee*), the fruit. It is the state of pure consciousness, or total bliss. All of the limbs of yoga lead to samadhi.

## Your Yoga Practice

Whether you're nine or ninety, you can enjoy and greatly benefit from practicing yoga. Its requirements are minimal. You need only 30 to 60 minutes each day; a nonskid mat; comfortable, nonrestrictive clothing; and a small exercise space. Turn off your phone, put on the answering machine, and let your family and friends know that you're not to be disturbed during your yoga time—unless, of course, they want to join you. You'll be able to create your own yoga weight loss home practice by following the yoga programs presented in Chapter 2, "Before You Begin"; Chapter 3, "Yoga Power Workout"; Chapter 4, "Yoga for Abdominals"; Chapter 5, "Yoga for Toning"; Chapter 6, "Gentle Yoga"; and Chapter 7, "Yoga Food."

You'll notice that the practice workouts in this book include poses that stretch the spine in six directions. In yoga there is a saying, "You're as young as your spine." If you stretch your spine in six directions during your daily practice you will be richly rewarded with a youthful, flexible, strong back and body. The six directions (and some representative postures) are

- Forward (Standing Forward Bend)
- Backward (Standing Backbend)
- Right side (Standing Side-to-Side Right)
- Left side (Standing Side-to-Side Left)
- Right twist (Seated Twist Right)
- Left twist (Seated Twist Right)

Every yoga workout ends with a relaxation period (see Chapter 6, "Gentle Yoga"). As you progress in your yoga study, you will also want to add meditation and breathing exercises (see Chapter 2, "Before You Begin," and Chapter 4, "Yoga for Abdominals"). As I mentioned earlier, yoga is a noncompetitive practice. There's no need to compete with other yogis or yoginis. Simply do the best that you can each and every time you practice. Your body will respond differently to the postures from day to day because of various factors, such as your diet, the amount of sleep you've had, and the time of day you're practicing. It is important to remember that the practice of yoga is a journey and an exploration into the nature of your self.

Practicing yoga is well worth it. Believe it, do it, and see it. There's nothing to it but to do it! Then you'll lose it—weight, that is—as you gain strength, beauty, flexibility, and good health. *Namaste!* (*Namaste* is a traditional yoga blessing that means "The divine in me bows to the divine in you.")

## Your Yoga for Weight Loss Program

The Yoga for Weight Loss Program includes four workout steps to help you lose weight and get in shape in the shortest time possible. Begin with Step 1 and continue with Steps 2 through 4, according to your physical condition and capabilities. An overview of each step and workout plan follows. You can find a more detailed description of each workout plan in Chapters 2 through 6.

Step 1: The Yoga Basics and Gentle Yoga Workout Plan

Step 2: Yoga Power Workout Plans (Beginner, Beginner-Intermediate, Intermediate, Intermediate-Advanced, and Maintenance)

Step 3: The 10-Minute Yoga for Abs Workout

Step 4: The Yoga Toning Practice Plan

## STEP 1. YOGA BASICS AND GENTLE YOGA WORKOUT PLAN

Begin with the Yoga Basics and Gentle Yoga Workout poses found in Chapters 2 and 6, and practice for 2 weeks. Do these poses for 30 minutes, 3 or 4 days a week. Each practice session includes Warm Up, Postures practice, and a Cool Down/Relaxation period. Be aware that it may take you more than 2 weeks to do this routine comfortably, depending on your physical condition. If you feel comfortable and confident doing these poses, proceed to the Yoga Power Workouts. Otherwise, stay with Weeks 1 and 2 until you feel strong enough to continue. See Chapters 2 and 6 for the detailed workout.

## STEP 2. YOGA POWER WORKOUT PLANS

After about 2 weeks of Yoga Basics and Gentle Yoga, select one of the five 4-week Yoga Power Workouts in Chapter 3—Beginner, Beginner-Intermediate, Intermediate, Intermediate-Advanced, or Maintenance. These Yoga Power Workouts will help you lose weight and get in shape in the shortest time possible. Each practice session includes Warm Up, Yoga Power and/or aerobics exercises, and a Cool

Down/Relaxation period. As you progress from Beginner to Maintenance over a period of 4 months and beyond, you'll build your yoga practice up from 30 to 60 minutes a day, 3 to 6 days a week. See Chapter 3 for detailed workouts.

To burn additional calories and for an even more efficient workout, add Yoga Abdominals and Toning to your practice on alternate days (see the 10-Minute Yoga for Abs Workout and the Yoga Toning Practice Plan), below.

### 1. Beginner Yoga Power Workout
### Weeks 1 through 4

Start with the Beginner Yoga Power Workout, combining Sun Salutation A and aerobics, 4 or 5 days a week for 30 to 40 minutes.

### 2. Beginner-Intermediate Yoga Power Workout
### Weeks 1 through 4

After completing the Beginner Yoga Power Workout, continue with the Beginner-Intermediate Yoga Power Workout, combining Sun Salutation B and aerobics, 4 or 5 days a week for 50 minutes.

### 3. Intermediate Yoga Power Workout
### Weeks 1 through 4

After completing the Beginner-Intermediate Yoga Power Workout, continue with the Intermediate Yoga Power Workout, combining Sun Salutation C and aerobics, 5 days a week for 50 to 60 minutes.

### 4. Intermediate-Advanced Yoga Power Workout
### Weeks 1 through 4

After completing the Intermediate Yoga Power Workout, continue with the Intermediate-Advanced Yoga Power Workout, combining Sun Salutation D, Moon Salutation, and aerobics, 5 or 6 days a week for 50 to 60 minutes.

### 5. Maintenance Yoga Power Workout
### Week 1 and Beyond

After completing the Intermediate-Advanced Yoga Power Workout, continue with the Maintenance Yoga Power Workout, combining Sun Salutation A, B, C, or D, Moon Salutation, and aerobics, 5 days a week for 50 to 60 minutes.

## STEP 3. 10-MINUTE YOGA FOR ABS WORKOUT

This 4-week yoga workout for abdominals can be practiced alone or in conjunction with the Yoga Power Workouts and Yoga Toning Practice. Do these poses for 10 minutes a day, 3 days a week. Be aware that it may take you more than 4 weeks to do this routine comfortably, depending on your physical condition. See Chapter 4 for the detailed workout.

## STEP 4. YOGA TONING PRACTICE PLAN

This 4-week Yoga Toning Workout can be practiced alone or combined with the Yoga Power Workouts and Yoga for Abs. Do the poses for 10 minutes, 2 or 3 days a week. Be aware that it may take you more than 4 weeks to do this routine comfortably, depending on your physical condition. See Chapter 5 for the detailed workout.

chapter 2

# Before You Begin

Before you begin your Yoga for Weight Loss Program you need to be aware of some cautions, as well as your weight loss goals. You can then begin your weight loss program with Step 1, the Yoga Basics and Gentle Yoga Workout Plan.

## A Word of Caution

Yoga should never cause you pain. Due to the intense stretching in some of the yoga poses, you need to be tuned in to your body. You should be aware of and realistic about where your "edge" is in each pose—the point beyond which your body can't comfortably go any further. Being at your edge should never cause a burning feeling of pain. As you explore each yoga pose, go slowly and cautiously, finding the point to which you can stretch safely. As you gradually become stronger and more flexible, you'll find that your edge will change. You'll be able comfortably and safely to stretch further and hold the poses longer.

Before beginning any new exercise program, you should always consult with your health care practitioner, especially if you have health problems or physical limitations. Also, women should be aware that practicing inverted postures, such as Half Shoulderstand and Legs-up-the-Wall Pose, is not recommended during the first few days of menstruation. If you are pregnant, be sure to obtain clearance from your physician before beginning a hatha yoga program. There are many excellent prenatal yoga classes with certified instructors that teach specific prenatal yoga routines.

Never practice yoga poses that cause you pain or discomfort. If pain persists, be sure to consult with your health care professional.

## Your Weight Loss Goals

Before beginning this yoga program, try to be clear about your weight loss goals. How much weight do you think you need to lose? Is your goal to fit into clothing two sizes smaller? How realistic is that?

Set reachable and reasonable goals and know that it will take some time to reach them.

One way to help set your weight loss goals and monitor your progress is to calculate your Body Mass Index (BMI). Obesity is defined as being 20 to 30 pounds above the average weight for your age, sex, and height and having a BMI of over 30. The BMI is a height-weight calculation that correlates body fat with risk for disease. According to the National Institutes of Health, the BMI is a better measure of obesity than just body weight and helps identify your risk of developing health problems such as heart disease, Type 2 diabetes, and high blood pressure.

To figure out your BMI, multiply your weight in pounds by 700. Then divide this number by the square of your height in inches. A BMI between 20 and 25 is considered a healthy number for men and women. A BMI over 25 suggests that losing weight would be good for your health, and a BMI of less than 19 indicates you're most likely underweight.

For example, if you're 20 pounds above the average weight for your age, sex, and height and have a BMI of 27, a reachable goal may be to lose 10 pounds. If losing 10 pounds reduces your BMI to under 25, you will then want to set a goal to maintain your healthy body weight by eating nutritious meals and continuing your yoga practice. However, if your BMI remains at 25 or over, you may want to set another goal to lose 5 to 10 more pounds.

Another way to measure body fat and health risk is to calculate your waist-to-hip ratio—the distribution of body weight around your midsection. Excess abdominal fat (an apple shape), independent of total body weight, indicates increased health risks. To calculate your own waist-to-hip ratio, measure your waist at the navel, and your hips at the widest point around the buttocks. Divide your waist size by your hip size. A result over 0.75 in women or 0.85 in men indicates an increased health risk.

Your waist circumference can also indicate foreseeable yet preventable health risks. If you are a woman with a waist measurement over 35 inches or a man whose waist exceeds 40 inches, you are at a higher risk to develop diabetes, hypertension, and cardiovascular disease. However, merely being thin does not necessarily mean a person is healthy and fit. What's most important for good health are your cardiovascular fitness, flexibility, and strength.

How much time are you allowing yourself to reach your weight loss goals? It usually takes a minimum of 2 to 3 months of consistent yoga exercise, nutritious meals, and eating modifications (see Chapter 7, "Yoga Food") before changes in strength, flexibility, and body composition (less fat and more muscle) begin to appear. Depending on your physical condition when you began this yoga program, it may take 6 months or more before your body really starts to show results. You may want to begin a yoga journal and jot down your thoughts about how you look and feel, to help yourself pinpoint areas you would like to change.

It's a good idea to check your progress every 3 months and reevaluate your goals. For example, after 3 months of following the Yoga Power Workout Plans in Chapter 3, you may be finishing the Intermediate Yoga Power Workout. At this point, you will want to measure your BMI and your waist-to-hip ratio and see if there are any changes. Depending on these results and your comfort level during the workout, you may want a higher intensity routine, and so you may advance to the Intermediate-Advanced Yoga Power Workout.

Individuals who combine hefty food portions and caloric intake with inactive lives sitting in front of computers and televisions, taking elevators instead of walking up the stairs, and driving from office to home make it easy to see why ninety-seven million Americans are overweight. Many of us need to bring daily physical activity and nutritious eating back into our lives. Please keep in mind that the Yoga for Weight Loss Program is not only workouts, it's a lifestyle modification program designed to establish good habits to improve and protect your health and appearance. Make a daily affirmation to yourself to reach your weight loss goals through yoga exercise and healthy eating.

## Yoga Basics

An understanding of certain fundamental movements will help you to perform the yoga postures in this book correctly. The following basic yoga preparations are incorporated into many yoga postures and will help you build strength, flexibility, and proper alignment in your upper body and lower back.

The squeeze, hold, and release actions found in Shoulder Press and Squeeze and Pelvic Tilt are fundamental to yoga practice, massaging tension and stress out of a particular area while bringing fresh, oxygenated blood into the muscles and tissues. Lifting the sternum (see Mountain Pose, page 27) is repeated over and over again within many yoga postures.

The use of your core strength—the lifting of your abdominals for maximum support—is also essential while performing yoga postures. In yoga, this includes the *mula bandha*, or "root lock," which contracts the perineum (see page 31) and the *uddiyana bandha*, which contracts the abdomen (see page 114). The mula bandha and uddiyana bandha actions are incorporated into the yoga poses and draw awareness to the core of your body. These contractions build a strong foundation in your body and strengthen the abdominal, pelvic, and genital muscles.

*Ujjayi* breathing is a classic *pranayama* (yoga breathing) technique. It can be joined with Sun Salutation asanas (pages 55 to 85) to help link the postures together and energize your practice. After yoga practice it's important to relax deeply in a Relaxation Pose, or Savasana (pages 168 and 170), and practice Observation Meditation (page 32) for a few minutes to enhance the effectiveness of the poses and calm the mind and nervous system.

## The Yoga Basics and Gentle Yoga Workout Plan

Begin your first 2 weeks of yoga practice with the following Yoga Basics poses and the Gentle Yoga poses you will find in Chapter 6. Be aware that it may take you more than 2 weeks to do this routine comfortably, depending on your physical condition. If you feel comfortable and confident doing these poses, proceed to the Yoga Power Workouts found in Chapter 3. Otherwise, stay with Weeks 1 and 2 until your feel strong enough to continue.

## Week 1

**Workout Schedule:** Practice for 30 minutes, 3 or 4 times a week. Warm up with Yoga Basics poses, proceed to Gentle Yoga postures, and then cool down with a few more Yoga Basics poses.

**Warm Up:**
Shoulder Press and Squeeze
Pelvic Tilt
Mountain Pose and Lifting the Sternum
Chest Expander

**Gentle Yoga:**
Seated Forward Hang
Seated Wheel Pose
Seated Side-to-Side
Seated Twist
Seated Triangle Pose
Seated Chest Expander

**Cool Down:**

Ujjayi Pranayama

Mula Bandha

Seated or Supported Relaxation Pose and Observation Meditation

## Week 2

**Workout Schedule:** Practice for 30 to 40 minutes, 4 times a week. Warm up with Yoga Basics poses, proceed to Gentle Yoga poses, and then cool down with a few more Yoga Basics poses.

**Warm Up:**

Shoulder Press and Squeeze

Pelvic Tilt

Mountain Pose and Lifting the Sternum

Chest Expander

**Gentle Yoga:**

Modified Spread-Leg Forward Bend

Modified Tree Pose

Modified Warrior I Pose

Modified Warrior III Pose

Legs-up-the-Wall Pose

Modified Child's Pose
Modified Reclining Big Toe Pose

**Cool Down:**
Ujjayi Pranayama
Mula Bandha
Seated or Supported Relaxation Pose and Observation Meditation

## Yoga Basics Poses

### SHOULDER PRESS AND SQUEEZE

**What It Does:** These shoulder movements are incorporated into many yoga postures, including Dolphin Headstand Preparation (page 135), Cobra (page 57), Downward-Facing Dog (page 84), Supported Relaxation Pose (page 168), Inclined Plane (page 137), Bound Lunge (page 133) and Chest Expander (page 29). These squeeze, hold, and release actions are fundamental to yoga practice, massaging tension and stress out of a particular area while bringing fresh, oxygenated blood into the muscles and tissues.

**How to Do It:**

1. Sit up straight on the mat with your legs crossed, arms at your sides.

2. Inhale and raise your shoulders toward your ears. Squeeze and hold for 4 counts. Exhale and release, pressing your shoulders down and away from your ears.

3. Clasp your hands behind your back. Inhale and straighten your elbows. Press your shoulders down and away from your ears. Exhale and gently squeeze your shoulder blades together. Hold for 3 counts. Release your hands.

4. Repeat.

## MOUNTAIN POSE AND LIFTING THE STERNUM (*TADASANA*)

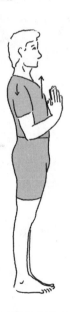

**What It Does:** The subtle but important action of lifting the sternum or breastbone toward the ceiling is incorporated into many yoga postures, including Standing Backbend (page 55) and Seated Forward Bend (page 107).

### How to Do It:

1. Stand in Mountain Pose: feet together, legs straight, and hands in prayer position over your heart center. Visualize a string attached to your sternum or breastbone (the bone in the center of your chest).

2. Inhale and visualize the string being pulled up toward the ceiling. Feel the subtle lifting and expanding of your chest, rib cage, and sternum, lengthening the front of your body. Keep your shoulders relaxed and down, away from your ears.

3. Exhale and release.

4. Repeat.

## PELVIC TILT

**What It Does:** These pelvic movements are incorporated into many yoga postures, including Standing Backbend (page 55), Bridge Pose (page

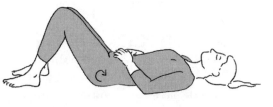

110). Single Leg Lifts (page 104), and Cobra (page 57). The lower-back press, hold, and release actions are fundamental movements in yoga, massaging tension and stress away while bringing fresh, oxygenated blood into the muscles and tissues. It is essential to tighten the buttock muscles firmly to protect and stabilize your lower back and activate the abdominals.

**How to Do It:**

1. Lie on your back on the mat, knees bent and feet flat on the mat, hip-width apart. Rest your hands on your abdomen. Inhale and allow your lower back to arch naturally.

2. Exhale, tightening your buttock muscles, tilting your pelvis under, and pulling your abdomen in. Press the small of your back gently to the mat. Inhale and release.

3. Repeat.

## CHEST EXPANDER

**What It Does:** This exercise incorporates all three movements that came before: the Shoulder Press and Squeeze, Pelvic Tilt, and Mountain Pose and Lifting the Sternum. If your shoulders and chest are tight, try clasping a towel or belt behind you while doing this exercise.

**How to Do It:**

1. Stand with your feet hip-width apart and clasp your hands behind your back.

2. Inhale, lifting your sternum toward the ceiling as you press your shoulders down and away from your ears. Exhale, straightening your elbows and gently squeezing your shoulder blades together. Tighten the buttock muscles, tilt the pelvis under, and pull the abdomen in.

3. Inhale, release, and relax.

## UJJAYI PRANAYAMA

**What It Does:** Ujjayi breathing is a classic pranayama (yoga breathing) technique. It is joined with Sun Salutation (pages 55 to 85) to help link the postures together and energize your practice.

**How to Do It:**

1. Keeping your lips closed, constrict the back of your throat, or the glottis (the opening between the vocal chords), during inhalation and exhalation. This produces a hissing sound, like that heard at the approach of Darth Vader.

2. If this is too difficult, try to whisper the sound "aaah" while inhaling and exhaling through your open mouth.

3. Close your lips and breathe through your nose, continuing to make the hissing or "aaah" sound at the back of your throat.

## MULA BANDHA

**What It Does:** The mula bandha, or "root lock," contracts the perineum, or pelvic floor, which comprises the pubococcygeus muscles between the rectum and genitals. This draws awareness to the core of your body, builds a strong foundation in your body, and strengthens the abdominal, pelvic, and genital muscles.

**How to Do It:**

1. Sit on a chair or cross-legged on the floor, sitting straight and tall. To visualize where your pelvic muscles are, imagine stopping the flow of your urine. Inhale, then exhale and contract these muscles, pulling up through your genital area and drawing up through your spine. Inhale and release the muscles.

2. Isolate the muscle group around your anus. Inhale, then exhale, contracting them and drawing them upward. Inhale and release the muscles.

3. Now combine the two actions. Inhale, then exhale and contract the muscles of your anus and genitals at the same time. Inhale and release the muscles.

## OBSERVATION MEDITATION

**What It Does:** Yoga Observation Meditation practices *svadhyaya* (the understanding of self), which is part of niyama, one of the eight limbs of Yoga as described in Patanjali's *Yoga Sutras* (see Chapter 1). This practice includes self-observation, which nurtures introspection, serenity, and cosmic connectedness, ultimately leading to a universal union with all that you are.

**How to Do It:**

1. Sit straight in a chair with your legs together and feet flat on the floor, or lie down in Supported Relaxation Pose (page 168). Be sure that you're comfortable and relaxed in this position.

2. Applying self-observation helps you discover and sense changes in your body and mind. For several minutes or longer, sense the changes going on in your body externally and internally. Observe how you're feeling. How does your skin feel? Does it tingle? Is it warm? After your yoga stretches, sense and enjoy the energy and

warmth flowing to areas that were previously stiff with tension or fatigued. Consciously try to relax any areas that still have tension, fatigue, or pain.

3. Calmly take note of the flow of your thoughts. Is your mind restless? Do you have negative thoughts and suggestions? Quiet your mind by focusing on your breath. Center your attention on the tip of your nose. Observe the coolness of the air as it flows into your nostrils, and the warmth of the air as it flows out. Hold your attention on your breath. If your mind wanders, simply bring it back to the breath as it flows in and out of your nostrils. Be in the moment.

4. Now replace your negative thoughts with positive suggestions, such as uplifting words, affirmations, thoughts, and prayers. Breathe in love, light, energy, and healing to every cell of your body. Breathe out all negativity, darkness, tension, and fatigue. Rest your body and mind for as long as you like. Practice this simple meditation daily to nourish your body, mind, and spirit.

# Yoga Power Workout

Want to melt off pounds, increase your strength and flexibility, stretch your spiritual muscles, and find inner peace at the same time? You can achieve all that and more with a combination of yoga and aerobics by following the Yoga Power Workout, which will burn loads of calories, raise your metabolism, and promote your cardiovascular health. Over the years, I've seen how powerfully effective a combination workout of yoga and aerobics can be. This workout is the most efficient way to lose weight or maintain your ideal weight, and it allows you to make the most out of your workout time.

At first glance, yoga and aerobics may appear to lie on opposite ends of the fitness spectrum, but in actuality they complement each other. Yoga and aerobics are the perfect yin and yang of strength and flexibility. The aerobics part of the workout burns calories, raises the heart rate and metabolism, and creates heat, which in turn augments the Power Yoga segment of the workout and melts off more pounds, as it strengthens and stretches the muscles and calms the mind.

To condition your heart and lungs, boost your metabolism, and burn calories while reducing your risk of heart disease, cancer, and diabetes, medical experts recommend doing aerobic workouts, such as brisk walking, easy jogging, running, treadmill walking/jogging, swimming, step aerobics, stationary cycling, or jumping rope, 3 or 4 times a week for 30 to 40 minutes. One of the misconceptions about yoga is that it doesn't provide enough of a cardiovascular workout. However, a vigorous *ashtanga vinyasa*, or power yoga, practice can be just as effective as many aerobic activities.

Ashtanga yoga practice consists primarily of vinyasas, or continuous flows of poses. One pose follows another so that you're constantly moving between the poses without resting. This results in a superlative cardiovascular workout that challenges your flexibility, strength, and endurance. Combining aerobics and ashtanga yoga increases cardiovascular intensity, and it is a fantastic way to burn calories and sculpt your buns.

## Weight Loss Basics

You've been on a low-calorie diet and you work out twice a week, but you still can't lose those last few pounds. Sound familiar? Many of us blame weight gain on our slow metabolisms, but the fact is, most of us have normal metabolisms that are neither too slow nor too fast. That doesn't mean you can't change yours. You can, and for the better. Here's how: exercise.

To lose weight, you must burn more calories than you consume. You can increase your metabolism and the number of calories you burn by increasing the amount that you exercise. For losing weight, fitness experts recommend regular aerobic exercise, such as the Yoga Power Workouts that follow.

To lose 1 pound, you need to burn 3,500 calories. If you can create a deficit of 500 calories each day for 7 days, then at the end of the week you'll have lost 1 pound. You don't have to be a math whiz to figure out that if you stick with it, you can lose as much as 52 pounds in a year. Working out smarter, not necessarily harder, is one of the keys to increasing your metabolism and losing weight. Since muscles adapt and become more metabolically efficient with the same workout, you need to vary your yoga and aerobic routine periodically to challenge your muscles and cardiovascular system. The 4-week Yoga Power routines I've created do just that.

## Turn Up the Calorie Burn

Another way for you to burn more calories than usual and boost your metabolism is to incorporate interval training into your Yoga Power sessions. Interval training increases the heart rate, training intensity, and caloric burning by adding 1-minute periods of more intense, anaerobic exercises to your aerobic program. Vigorous exercise such as walking, running, or cycling, performed continuously for longer than 3 or 4 minutes, is considered aerobic exercise. Performing all-out exercise, such as in sprinting, weight-lifting, or climbing, in short bursts—up to 60 seconds—is considered anaerobic exercise.

Aerobic and anaerobic exercise will burn calories derived from carbohydrates and fat. Aerobic exercise, such as running or walking for more than 20 minutes at 65 percent of your maximum heart rate (MHR), allows your body to use fat as a source of fuel (see the following section). This is your fat-burning zone. You will burn fat and lose weight if you continue to exercise at this aerobic intensity 6 to 7 times a week for 50 to 60 minutes, as you will if you follow the Yoga

Power Workouts below. Engaging in high-intensity, anaerobic exercise at 85 to 100 percent of MHR for up to 60 seconds will burn primarily carbohydrate calories, thereby allowing you to burn more calories during the course of the day.

To increase calorie-burning intensity, try the Intermediate, Intermediate-Advanced, and Maintenance Yoga Power Workouts, which incorporate 1-minute interval training into your Yoga Power routine. Within 24 hours after your workout, your metabolism will rev faster, burning a few hundred more calories than usual. Be forewarned, interval training is not for beginners. However, as your level of fitness increases, you will increase your strength and endurance, as well as your ability to incorporate and benefit from interval training.

## FAT/CARBS BURNING ZONES

1. To find your maximum heart rate, subtract your age from 220. For example, for a 20-year-old woman, $220 - 20 = 200$ beats per minute (BPM).

2. To determine the low end of your fat-burning zone, find 50 percent of your maximum heart rate. For example, $200 \text{ MHR} \times 0.5 =$

100. To determine the high end of your fat-burning zone, find 65 percent of your maximum heart rate. For example, 200 MHR × 0.65 = 130. This is for experienced exercisers. Beginners should work at the low end of the fat-burning zone. Gradually build up to the high end to reach your maximum fat-burning zone.

3. To determine your carbs-burning zone, find 90 percent of your maximum heart rate. For example, 200 MHR × 0.90 = 180. Only advanced exercisers should work out at this range.

4. To check your heart rate during sustained, aerobic exercise, place your index and middle fingers on the pulse point of your opposite wrist. Using a watch with a second hand, count the beats for 10 seconds. Multiply the number of beats by 6 to get your heart rate. Be sure your pulse stays within your range. Check your pulse periodically throughout your aerobic workout and immediately after finishing.

5. Always pay attention to your body's signals of overexertion, such as pounding in your chest, dizziness, faintness, profuse sweating, and an inability to carry on a normal conversation due to shortness of breath. If any of these symptoms occurs, you need to slow your pace. If symptoms persist, see your doctor.

## Before You Start

- If you're just beginning a fitness program, remember to work up to the recommended frequency and duration comfortably and gradually.
- Perform the vinyasas slowly, according to your own capacity. You should never be in pain, nor should you experience breathlessness.
- Always consult with your physician before beginning a new exercise program.

## Your 4-Week Yoga Power Workout

Select one of the following five Yoga Power Workout Plans to lose weight and get in shape in the shortest time possible. The vinyasas presented in this chapter include the Sun Salutation and three variations for different levels of experience, as well as the Moon Salutation. You can begin the Yoga Power Workout after practicing the Yoga Basics and Gentle Yoga Workouts found in chapters 2 and 6 for 2 weeks. Be aware that it may take you more than 2 weeks to do this routine comfortably, depending on your physical condition. If you feel comfortable and confident doing these poses, proceed to the Yoga Power Workout.

Begin with the simpler Yoga Power variations, which will help you build the stamina, strength, and coordination necessary to practice the more challenging ones. As you progress from Beginner to Maintenance over a period of 4 months and beyond, you'll build your yoga practice up from 30 to 60 minutes a day, 3 to 6 days a week.

While practicing the first vinyasa cycle, you may feel stiff and clumsy. By the second or third cycle, the movements will start flowing more easily and the rhythm of your breathing will become more natural.

As you practice the vinyasas, focus not only on each pose but also on the use of your breath. Breath links the postures together in vinyasa practice and energizes your aerobic exercise. During your Yoga Power Workout, maintain deep, rhythmic breathing, synchronizing the flow of yoga postures or aerobic movements with your inhalation and exhalation. A general guideline to follow is to inhale when doing backbends and exhale when doing forward-bending postures. Ujjayi breathing is a classic pranayama (yoga breathing) technique used especially during vinyasa. During ujjayi breathing you keep your breath steady and controlled (see page 23).

Vinyasa yoga's full-body workout and powerful combination of stretching with strength and balance will produce beneficial physical improvements within a short time. Your spine will become more supple, and tight hamstrings will begin to release, as you tone, firm, and strengthen your body.

## Yoga Power Workout Plans

### 1. BEGINNER YOGA POWER WORKOUT PLAN

After practicing the Yoga Basics and Gentle Yoga Workouts found in chapters 2 and 6 for 2 weeks, beginners should start with Sun Salutation A. After you've finished this 4-week Beginner plan, you can proceed to the Beginner-Intermediate Yoga Power Workout Plan. But be aware that it may take you more than 4 weeks to do this routine comfortably, depending on your physical condition. Feel free to take as much time as you need before progressing to Beginner-Intermediate practice.

To burn additional calories and make your workout even more efficient, add Yoga for Abs and Yoga Toning to your practice on alternate days (see Chapters 4 and 5).

## Weeks 1 and 2

**Workout Schedule:** Practice Sun Salutation A (page 55) 3 or 4 days a week for 20 to 30 minutes. On the remaining days of the week take a 15-minute walk, pacing yourself at 50 percent of your maximum heart rate.

**Warm Up:** Before beginning your repetitions of Sun Salutation A or walking, perform Sun Salutation A once slowly, holding each posture for 5 breaths.

**Sun Salutation A:** Perform 4 to 6 repetitions of Sun Salutation A, holding each posture for 3 breaths. Pace yourself at 50 percent of your maximum heart rate (see the "Fat/Carbs Burning Zones" section, page 39).

**Aerobics:** Walk for 15 minutes, pacing yourself at 50 percent of your maximum heart rate.

**Cool Down:** Perform 1 repetition of Sun Salutation A slowly, holding each posture for 5 breaths. End with 5 to 10 minutes of Supported Relaxation Pose.

## Weeks 3 and 4

**Workout Schedule:** Practice Sun Salutation A 4 or 5 days a week for 30 minutes, followed by a 15-minute walk.

**Warm Up:** Perform Sun Salutation A once slowly, holding each posture for 5 breaths.

**Sun Salutation A:** Perform 6 to 8 repetitions of Sun Salutation A with increasing speed, holding each posture for 1 to 3 breaths. Pace yourself at 50 to 65 percent of your maximum heart rate.

**Aerobics:** Walk for 15 minutes, pacing yourself at 50 to 65 percent of your maximum heart rate.

**Cool Down:** Perform 1 repetition of Sun Salutation A slowly, holding each posture for 5 breaths. End with 5 to 10 minutes of Supported Relaxation Pose (page 168).

## 2. BEGINNER-INTERMEDIATE YOGA POWER WORKOUT PLAN

Once you've mastered Sun Salutation A, you can progress to Sun Salutation B. After you've finished this 4-week Beginner-Intermediate plan, you can proceed to the Intermediate Yoga Power Workout. But be aware that it may take you more than 4 weeks to do this routine comfortably, depending on your physical condition. Feel free to take as much time as you need before progressing to Intermediate practice.

To burn additional calories and make your workout even more efficient, you can incorporate Yoga for Abs and Yoga Toning, as described in Chapters 4 and 5, into your practice.

## Weeks 1 and 2

**Workout Schedule:** Practice Sun Salutation B (page 60) 4 or 5 days a week for 30 minutes, followed by a 20-minute walk.

**Warm Up:** Perform Sun Salutation A once slowly, holding each posture for 5 breaths.

**Sun Salutation B:** Perform 4 to 6 repetitions of Sun Salutation B, holding each posture for 3 breaths. Pace yourself at 50 to 65 percent of your maximum heart rate.

**Aerobics:** Walk briskly for 20 minutes, pacing yourself at 50 to 65 percent of your maximum heart rate.

**Cool Down:** Perform 1 repetition of Sun Salutation A slowly, holding each posture for 5 breaths. End with 5 to 10 minutes of Supported Relaxation Pose.

## Weeks 3 and 4

**Workout Schedule:** Practice Sun Salutation B 5 days a week for 30 minutes, followed by 20 minutes of aerobic activity.

**Warm Up:** Perform Sun Salutation A once slowly, holding each posture for 5 breaths.

**Sun Salutation B:** Perform 6 to 8 repetitions of Sun Salutation B with increasing speed, holding each posture for 1 to 3 breaths. Pace yourself at 50 to 65 percent of your maximum heart rate.

**Aerobics:** Instead of walking, do a different aerobic activity, such as easy jogging or stationary cycling, for 20 minutes. Pace yourself at 50 to 65 percent of your maximum heart rate.

**Cool Down:** Perform 1 repetition of Sun Salutation A slowly, holding each posture for 5 breaths. End with 5 to 10 minutes of Supported Relaxation Pose.

## 3. INTERMEDIATE YOGA POWER WORKOUT PLAN

Once you've mastered Sun Salutations A and B, you can progress to Sun Salutation C (page 66). After you've finished this 4-week Intermediate plan, you can proceed to the Intermediate-Advanced Yoga Power Workout. But be aware that it may take you more than 4 weeks to do this routine comfortably, depending on your physical condition. Feel free to take as much time as you need before progressing to Intermediate-Advanced practice.

To burn additional calories and for an even more efficient workout, you can incorporate Yoga for Abs and Yoga Toning, as described in Chapters 4 and 5, into your practice.

## Weeks 1 and 2

**Workout Schedule:** Practice Sun Salutation C 5 days a week for 30 minutes, followed by 20 minutes of your favorite aerobic activity, such as walking, easy jogging, treadmill walking/jogging, or stationary cycling.

**Warm Up:** Perform Sun Salutation A once slowly, holding each posture for 5 breaths.

**Sun Salutation C:** Perform 4 to 6 repetitions of Sun Salutation C, holding each posture for 3 breaths. Pace yourself at 50 to 65 percent of your maximum heart rate.

**Aerobics:** 20 minutes of your preferred aerobic activity plus 3 intervals, 1 minute each, of higher-intensity activity. For example, if you've chosen walking for your aerobic component, walk 5 minutes, then speed-walk or jog for 1 minute; repeat the sequence 2 times and walk for the remaining 5 minutes. If you're jogging, then sprint for 1-minute intervals; if you're stationary cycling, add 1-minute intervals of jumping rope; if you're treadmill walking, increase your speed or incline. Pace yourself at 50 to 65 percent of your maximum heart rate.

**Cool Down:** Perform 1 repetition of Sun Salutation A slowly, holding each posture for 5 breaths. End with 5 to 10 minutes of Supported Relaxation Pose.

## Weeks 3 and 4

**Workout Schedule:** Practice Sun Salutation C 5 days a week for 30 minutes, followed by 30 minutes of aerobic activity.

**Warm Up:** Perform Sun Salutation A once slowly, holding each posture for 5 breaths.

**Sun Salutation C:** Perform 6 to 8 repetitions of Sun Salutation C with increasing speed, holding each posture for 1 to 3 breaths. Pace yourself at 50 to 65 percent of your maximum heart rate.

**Aerobics:** 30 minutes of your preferred aerobic activity plus 4 intervals, 1 minute each, of higher-intensity activity. For example, if you're walking, walk 5 minutes, then speed-walk or do an easy jog for 1 minute; repeat the sequence 3 times and walk for the remaining 10 minutes. If you're jogging, then sprint during the 1-minute intervals; if you're stationary cycling, add 1-minute intervals of jumping rope; if you're treadmill walking, increase your speed or incline. Pace yourself at 50 to 65 percent of your maximum heart rate.

**Cool Down:** Perform 1 repetition of Sun Salutation A slowly, holding each posture for 5 breaths. End with 5 to 10 minutes of Supported Relaxation Pose.

## 4. INTERMEDIATE–ADVANCED YOGA POWER WORKOUT PLAN

Now that you've mastered Sun Salutations A, B, and C, you can progress to Sun Salutation D (page 71) and Moon Salutation (page 85). After you've finished this 4-week Intermediate plan, you can proceed to the Maintenance Yoga Power Workout. But be aware that it may take you more than 4 weeks to do this routine comfortably, depending on your physical condition. Feel free to take as much time as you need before progressing to Maintenance practice.

To burn additional calories and make your workout even more efficient, you can incorporate Yoga for Abs and Yoga Toning, as described in chapters 4 and 5, into your practice.

## Weeks 1 and 2

**Workout Schedule:** Practice Sun Salutation D and Moon Salutation 5 days a week for 30 minutes, followed by 30 minutes of your favorite aerobic activity, such as walking, easy jogging, treadmill walking/jogging, or stationary cycling.

**Warm Up:** Perform Sun Salutation A once slowly, holding each posture for 5 breaths.

**Sun Salutation D and Moon Salutation:** Perform Sun Salutation D once, and then perform Moon Salutation once, holding each posture for 3 breaths. Pace yourself at 50 to 65 percent of your maximum heart rate.

**Aerobics:** 30 minutes of aerobic activity plus 4 intervals, 1 minute each, of higher-intensity activity. For example, if you're walking, walk 5 minutes, then speed-walk or do an easy jog for 1 minute; repeat the sequence 3 times and continue walking for the remainder of the time. If you're jogging, then sprint during the 1-minute intervals; if you're stationary cycling, add 1-minute intervals of jumping rope; if you're treadmill walking, increase your speed or incline. Pace yourself at 50 to 65 percent of your maximum heart rate.

**Cool Down:** Perform 1 repetition of Sun Salutation A slowly, holding each posture for 5 breaths. End with 5 to 10 minutes of Supported Relaxation Pose.

## Weeks 3 and 4

**Workout Schedule:** Practice Sun Salutation D and Moon Salutation 6 days a week for 30 minutes, followed by 30 minutes of aerobic activity.

**Warm Up:** Perform Sun Salutation A once slowly, holding each posture for 5 breaths.

**Sun Salutation D and Moon Salutation:** Perform Sun Salutation D once, and then perform 2 repetitions of Moon Salutation with increasing speed, holding each posture for 1 to 3 breaths. Pace yourself at 50 to 65 percent of your maximum heart rate.

**Aerobics:** 30 minutes of aerobic activity plus 5 intervals, 1 minute each, of higher-intensity activity. For example, if you're walking, alternate 5 minutes of walking with 1-minute intervals of speed walking or an easy jog. If you're jogging, then sprint during the 1-minute intervals; if you're stationary cycling, add 1-minute intervals of jumping rope; if you're treadmill walking, increase your speed or incline. Pace yourself at 50 to 65 percent of your maximum heart rate.

**Cool Down:** Perform 1 repetition of Sun Salutation A slowly, holding each posture for 5 breaths. End with 5 to 10 minutes of Supported Relaxation Pose.

## 5. MAINTENANCE YOGA POWER WORKOUT PLAN

Congratulations! At this point, you've mastered Sun Salutations A, B, C, and D and Moon Salutation. I'm sure you're looking and feeling great. Follow the Maintenance Yoga Power Workout Plan to stay in shape and to continue to build and maintain your strength, cardiovascular fitness, and flexibility.

To burn additional calories and for an even more efficient workout, you can incorporate Yoga for Abs and Yoga Toning, as described in chapters 4 and 5, into your practice.

### Weeks 1 and Beyond

**Workout Schedule:** Alternate practice between Sun Salutations A, B, C, and D and Moon Salutation 5 days a week for 20 to 30 minutes, followed by 20 to 30 minutes of your favorite aerobic activity, such as walking, easy jogging, treadmill walking/jogging, or stationary cycling. If your schedule is busy, you can break up this routine. For example, you can practice Sun Salutation for 20 to 30 minutes in the morning and get your aerobic exercise at lunchtime with a brisk walk.

**Warm Up:** Perform Sun Salutation A once slowly, holding each posture for 5 breaths.

**Sun Salutation:** Perform 4 to 6 repetitions of Sun Salutation A, B, or C, or perform Sun Salutation D and Moon Salutation once each, with increasing speed, holding each posture for 1 to 3 breaths. Pace yourself at 50 to 65 percent of your maximum heart rate.

**Aerobics:** 20 to 30 minutes of aerobic activity plus 3 intervals, 1 minute each, of higher-intensity activity. For example, if you're walking, walk 5 minutes, then speed-walk or do an easy jog for 1 minute; repeat the sequence 2 times and continue walking for the remainder of the time. If you're jogging, then sprint during the 1-minute intervals; if you're stationary cycling, add 1-minute intervals of jumping rope; if you're treadmill walking, increase your speed or incline for 1 minute. Pace yourself at 50 to 65 percent of your maximum heart rate.

**Cool Down:** Perform Sun Salutation A once slowly, holding each posture for 5 breaths. End with 5 to 10 minutes of Supported Relaxation Pose (page 168).

## Yoga Vinyasas

## SUN SALUTATION A *(SURYA NAMASCAR VARIATION)*: BEGINNER AND WARM-UP

This ancient, classic yoga routine is traditionally done at sunrise but can of course be practiced any time of day, and is a complete workout for body and mind.

**1. Mountain Pose (*Tadasana*):** Stand with your feet together, legs straight, kneecaps tightened and pulled up, weight distributed evenly, and hands in prayer position over your heart center. Tilt your pelvis under, abdomen pulled in and shoulders relaxed and down, away from your ears. Lift your sternum toward the ceiling.

**2. Standing Backbend:** Inhale and raise your arms in a V overhead. Tighten your buttock muscles firmly to protect your lower back, lift your chest toward the ceiling, and bend backward. Pause for 3 seconds.

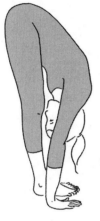

**3. Standing Forward Bend (*Uttanasana*):** Exhale, extending your arms forward, and fold your torso forward from the hips, abdomen in. Bend your knees slightly. Relax your face, head, neck, and shoulders toward the floor and lower your chest to your thighs. Place your hands on the floor, fingers in line with your toes.

**4. Left Lunge (*Anjaneyasana*):** Inhale, bending both knees and keeping your palms flat beside your feet. Step your right leg

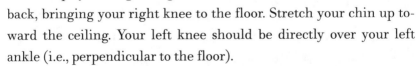

back, bringing your right knee to the floor. Stretch your chin up toward the ceiling. Your left knee should be directly over your left ankle (i.e., perpendicular to the floor).

**5. Plank Pose *(Chaturanga Dandasana)*:** Exhale, bringing your left leg back to join your right, and extend your arms, as you would to begin a push-up. Keep your body straight, legs and arms extended and head in line with spine. Pull your stomach in. Hold for 1 or 2 breaths.

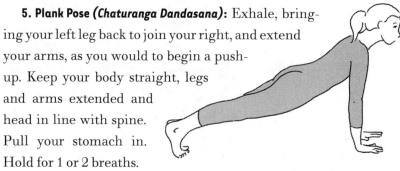

**6. Modified Plank Pose *(Modified Chaturanga Dandasana)*:** Exhale, bending and lowering knees, chest, and chin to the floor. Hips are up, abdomen is in. This pose is similar to a modified women's push-up. Keep your elbows close to your body. If this is too difficult, go from Plank Pose to placing the body flat, face down on the floor. Then go into a modified women's push-up position.

**7. Cobra *(Bhujangasana)*:** Inhale, raising forehead,

chin, and chest while arching your spine. Hips are on the floor. Elbows should be slightly bent and close to the body. Shoulders are pressed down and away from the ears. Tilt the pelvis under for lower-back protection. Pause for several breaths.

**8. Downward-Facing Dog (*Adho Mukha Svanasana*):** Exhale, lifting your hips up and back as you turn your body into an upside-down V. Keep your arms and legs straight and press your heels to the floor. Shoulders are pressed down and away from the ears.

**9. Right Lunge (*Anjaneyasana*):** Inhale, lunging your right foot forward between your two hands, toes in line with fingers. Look up, chin raised, palms flat, left knee on the floor.

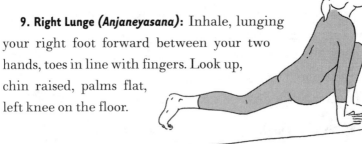

**10. Standing Forward Bend (*Uttanasana*):** Exhale, pushing off with the toes of your left foot to bring the left foot forward to join the right. Upper body is folded forward from the hips, knees are slightly bent, hands are on either side of the feet.

**11. Standing Backbend:** Inhale, raising yourself upright and keeping your back straight, your arms extended overhead and knees slightly bent. Exhale and tighten your buttocks. Inhale, keeping your head between your arms; lift the sternum toward the ceiling and arch your spine backward. Pause for 3 seconds.

**12. Mountain Pose (*Tadasana*):** Exhale; return to an upright position and bring your palms together. Take a few breaths, breathing in light and energy, exhaling tension and fatigue.

Repeat Steps 2 through 12 on the opposite leg, bringing the left leg back for Step 4, then forward for Step 9, for a complete cycle.

## SUN SALUTATION B
## (*SURYA NAMASCAR VARIATION*):
### BEGINNER-INTERMEDIATE

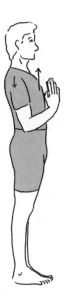

This variation is for the more advanced beginner and the intermediate-level practitioner.

**1. Mountain Pose (*Tadasana*):** Stand with your feet together, legs straight, kneecaps tightened and pulled up, weight distributed evenly and hands in prayer position over your heart center. Tilt your pelvis under, abdomen pulled in and shoulders relaxed and down, away from your ears. Lift your sternum toward the ceiling.

**2. Standing Side-to-Side (*Nitambasana*):**
Inhale, raising your arms up just behind your ears, your palms facing each other. Think of lifting your arms up and out of your rib cage. Exhale, stretching to the right. Pull your abdomen in. Come to center. Repeat left.

**3. Chest Expander Variation:**
Stand with your feet together, clasp your hands behind your back, and gently squeeze your shoulder blades together. Straighten your elbows, tightening your buttocks and knees. Inhale, expanding your chest and lifting your arms and chin. Exhale, folding forward from the hips, hands clasped above your head. Keep your legs as straight as possible. Bring your face toward your thighs. Slowly pull your arms to the right, then pull them to the left. Release your hands.

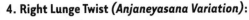

**4. Right Lunge Twist (*Anjaneyasana Variation*):**
Inhale, bending both knees, and place your palms flat on the mat beside your feet. Step your right foot back, bringing your right knee to the floor. Exhale; bring your torso upright, arms out to the sides in a T position. Inhale and twist shoulders to the right, looking over your right shoulder. Exhale, going back to your original position. Inhale, placing palms back down on either side of your left foot.

**5. Plank Pose (*Chaturanga Dandasana*):** Exhale, bringing your left leg back to join your right, and extend your arms, as if to begin a push-up. Keep your body straight, legs and arms extended and head in line with spine. Pull your abdomen in. Hold for several breaths.

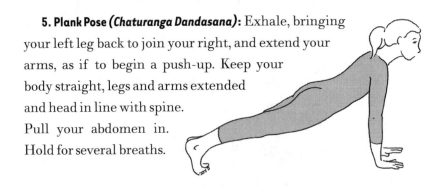

**6. Lowered Plank (Chaturanga Dandasana):** Exhale, bending your elbows and lowering

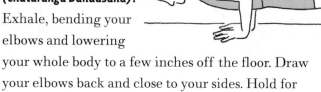

your whole body to a few inches off the floor. Draw your elbows back and close to your sides. Hold for 1 breath, then lower yourself to the floor.

**7. Cobra (Bhujangasana):** Inhale, raising your forehead, chin, and chest while arching your spine backward. Hips are on the floor. Your elbows should be slightly bent and close to your body. Shoulders are pressed down and away from your ears. Tilt the pelvis under for lower-back protection. Pause for several breaths.

**8. One-Legged Downward-Facing Dog (Adho Mukha Svanasana Variation):** Exhale, lifting your hips up and back and turning your body into an upside-down V. Keep your arms and legs straight and press your heels to the floor. Inhale, extend your left leg up toward the ceiling in line with your arms and spine, and press your right heel toward the floor. Exhale, bringing your leg back to the floor. Repeat with the right leg.

### 9. Left Lunge Prayer Twist (*Anjaneyasana Variation*):

Inhale, lunging your right foot forward between your two hands, toes in line with fingers. Exhale, lifting your chin, and gaze up. Palms are flat on the mat, left knee rests on the floor. Inhale; bring your torso upright, hands in prayer position. Exhale and twist your shoulders to the right, resting your left upper arm on your right knee. Inhale; look over your right shoulder. Exhale; return to your original position. Inhale, placing palms back on the mat on either side of your right foot.

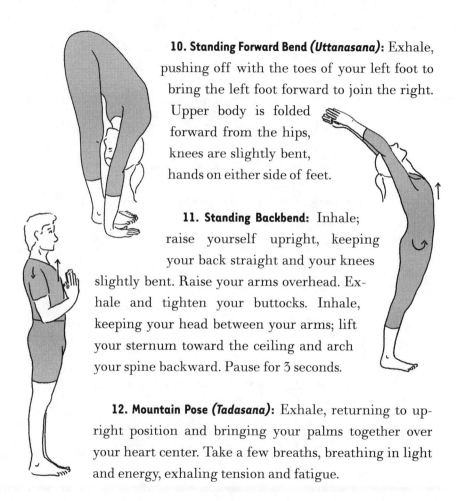

**10. Standing Forward Bend *(Uttanasana)*:** Exhale, pushing off with the toes of your left foot to bring the left foot forward to join the right. Upper body is folded forward from the hips, knees are slightly bent, hands on either side of feet.

**11. Standing Backbend:** Inhale; raise yourself upright, keeping your back straight and your knees slightly bent. Raise your arms overhead. Exhale and tighten your buttocks. Inhale, keeping your head between your arms; lift your sternum toward the ceiling and arch your spine backward. Pause for 3 seconds.

**12. Mountain Pose *(Tadasana)*:** Exhale, returning to upright position and bringing your palms together over your heart center. Take a few breaths, breathing in light and energy, exhaling tension and fatigue.

Repeat Steps 2 through 12 on the opposite leg, bringing your left leg back for Step 4, then forward for Step 9, for a complete cycle.

## SUN SALUTATION C
### *(SURYA NAMASCAR VARIATION)*: INTERMEDIATE

This power yoga variation is for the intermediate-level practitioner.

**1. Mountain Pose *(Tadasana)*:** Stand with your feet together, legs straight, kneecaps tightened and pulled up, weight distributed evenly, and hands in prayer position over your heart center. Tilt your pelvis under, abdomen pulled in and shoulders pulled down, away from your ears. Lift your sternum toward the ceiling.

**2. Standing Backbend:** Inhale and raise your arms in a V overhead. Tighten your buttock muscles firmly to protect your lower back, lift your chest toward the ceiling, and bend backward. Pause for 3 seconds.

**3. Standing Forward Bend (*Uttanasana*):** Exhale, extending your arms forward, and fold your torso forward from the hips, abdomen in. Bend your knees slightly. Relax your face, head, neck, and shoulders toward the floor and lower your chest to your thighs. Place your fingers on the floor in line with your toes.

**4. Monkey:** Inhale, extending your spine from the hips, and lift your head and chest away from your thighs. Roll your shoulders back and bend your knees if you need to.

**5. Standing Forward Bend (*Uttanasana*):** Exhale and fold your torso forward from the hips, abdomen in. Bend your knees slightly. Relax your face, head, neck, and shoulders toward the floor and lower your chest to your thighs.

**6. Plank Pose (Chaturanga Dandasana):** Exhale. Planting palms firmly on the mat, extend your right leg back, then your left. Extend your arms as if to begin a push-up. Keep your body straight, legs and arms extended and head in line with spine. Pull your stomach in. Hold for several breaths.

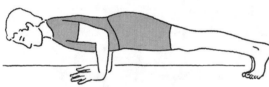

**7. Lowered Plank (Chaturanga Dandasana):** Exhale, bending your elbows and lowering your whole body to a few inches off the floor. Draw your elbows back and close to your sides. Hold for 1 breath, then lower yourself to the floor.

**8. Upward-Facing Dog (Urdhva Mukha Svanasana):** Inhale, pushing up with your arms and chest and arching your back, as in Cobra. Now lift your pelvis and legs slightly off the floor, resting your entire body weight on your hands and the tops of your feet. Draw your torso forward between straight arms and open your chest. Roll your shoulder blades down and keep your buttocks firm to protect your lower back. Abdomen is lifted.

**9. Downward-Facing Dog (*Adho Mukha Svanasana*):** Exhale, lifting your hips up and back as you turn your body into an upside-down V. Keep your arms and legs straight and press your heels to the floor. Shoulders are pressed down and away from the ears.

**10. Standing Forward Bend (*Uttanasana*):** Inhale, bring your right foot forward between your hands, then your left foot. Exhale, straightening your legs and folding your upper body forward from the hips.

**11. Monkey:** Inhale, extend your spine from the hips, and lift your head and chest away from your thighs. Roll your shoulders back and bend your knees if you need to.

**12. Standing Forward Bend (*Uttanasana*):** Exhale and fold your torso forward from the hips, abdomen in. Relax your face, head, neck, and shoulders toward the floor and lower your chest to your thighs.

**13. Mountain Pose (*Tadasana*):** Inhale, lifting your torso upright and keeping your back straight. Exhale, bringing your palms together in front of your heart center. Take a few breaths, breathing in light and energy, exhaling tension and fatigue.

## SUN SALUTATION D *(SURYA NAMASCAR VARIATION)*: INTERMEDIATE-ADVANCED

This variation incorporates Warrior II, Chair, and Triangle standing poses.

1. **Mountain Pose *(Tadasana)*:** Stand with your feet together, legs straight, kneecaps tightened and pulled up, weight distributed evenly, and hands in prayer position over your heart center. Tilt your pelvis under, abdomen pulled in and shoulders pulled down and away from the ears. Lift your sternum toward the ceiling.

2. **Standing Backbend:** Inhale and raise your arms in a V overhead. Tighten your buttock muscles firmly to protect your lower back, lift your chest toward the ceiling, and bend backward. Pause for 3 seconds.

**3. Standing Forward Bend (*Uttanasana*):** Exhale, extending your arms forward, and fold your torso forward from the hips, abdomen in. Bend your knees slightly. Relax your face, head, neck, and shoulders toward the floor and lower your chest to your thighs. Place your fingers on the floor in line with your toes.

**4. Monkey:** Inhale, extend your spine from the hips, and lift your head and chest away from your thighs. Roll your shoulders back and bend your knees if you need to.

**5. Standing Forward Bend (*Uttanasana*):** Exhale and fold your torso forward from the hips, abdomen in. Bend your knees slightly. Relax your face, head, neck, and shoulders toward the floor and lower your chest to your thighs.

**6. Raised Runner:** Inhale, bending both knees and placing your palms flat on the mat on either side of your feet. Step your right foot back, keeping your left leg bent. The right leg is straight, and the ball of the right foot is pressing into the floor.

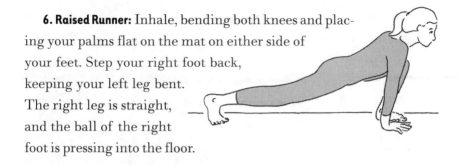

**7. Plank Pose (*Chaturanga Dandasana*):** Exhale, bringing your left leg back to join the right, as in a push-up position. Keep body straight, legs and arms extended and head in line with spine. Pull your abdomen in. Hold for several breaths.

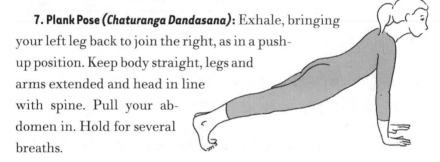

**8. Lowered Plank (*Chaturanga Dandasana*):** Exhale, bend your elbows, and lower your whole body to a few inches off

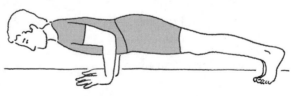

the floor. Draw your elbows back and close to your sides. Then lower yourself to the floor.

**9. Upward-Facing Dog (*Urdhva Mukha Svanasana*):** Inhale, pushing up with your arms and chest and arching your back, as in Cobra. Now lift your pelvis and legs slightly off the floor, resting your entire body weight on your hands and the tops of your feet. Draw your torso forward between straight arms and open your chest. Roll your shoulder blades down and keep your buttocks firm to protect your lower back. Abdomen is lifted.

**10. Downward-Facing Dog (*Adho Mukha Svanasana*):** Exhale, lifting your hips up and back as you turn your body into an upside-down V. Keep your arms and legs straight and press your heels to the floor. Shoulders are pressed down and away from the ears.

**11. Warrior II (*Virabhadrasana II*):** Exhale, lunging your right foot forward between your hands as you turn your left foot out to the side to rest flat. Inhale, lifting your torso and raising your arms out to the sides. Turn your hips and arms to the left, so that your hips are facing sideways, your right arm pointing forward and your left arm back. Bend your right knee to a 90-degree angle and turn your head to look toward your extended right fingertips. Inhale.

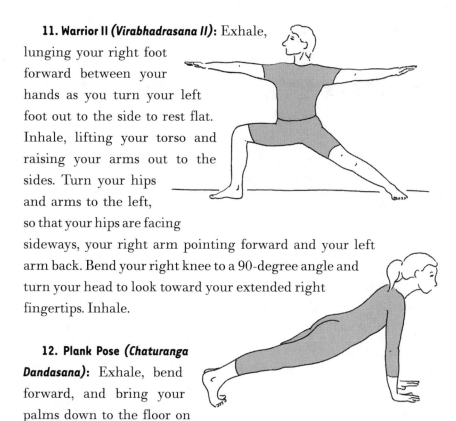

**12. Plank Pose (*Chaturanga Dandasana*):** Exhale, bend forward, and bring your palms down to the floor on either side of your right foot. Bring your right leg back to join your left and extend your arms, as if to start a push-up. Keep your body straight, legs and arms extended and head in line with spine. Pull your abdomen in.

**13. Lowered Plank (*Chaturanga Dandasana*):** Exhale, bend your elbows, and lower your whole body to a few inches off the floor. Draw your elbows back and close to your sides. Then lower yourself to the floor.

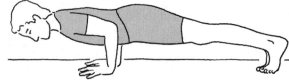

**14. Upward-Facing Dog (*Urdhva Mukha Svanasana*):** Inhale, pushing up with your arms and chest and arching your back, as in Cobra. Now lift your pelvis and legs slightly off the floor, resting your entire body weight on your hands and the tops of your feet. Draw your torso forward between straight arms and open your chest. Roll your shoulder blades down and keep your buttocks firm to protect your lower back. Abdomen is lifted.

### 15. Downward-Facing Dog *(Adho Mukha Svanasana)*:

Exhale, lifting the hips up and back as you turn your body into an upside-down V. Keep your arms and legs straight and press your heels to the floor. Shoulders are pressed down and away from the ears.

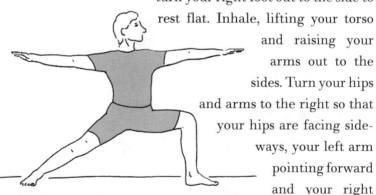

### 16. Warrior II *(Virabhadrasana II)*:

Exhale, lunging your left foot forward between your hands as you turn your right foot out to the side to rest flat. Inhale, lifting your torso and raising your arms out to the sides. Turn your hips and arms to the right so that your hips are facing sideways, your left arm pointing forward and your right arm back. Bend your left knee to a 90-degree angle and turn your head to look toward your extended left fingertips. Inhale.

**17. Plank Pose *(Chaturanga Dandasana)*:** Exhale, bend forward, and bring your palms down to the floor on either side of your right foot. Bring your right leg back to join the left and extend your arms, as if to start a push-up. Keep your body straight, legs and arms extended and head in line with spine. Pull your abdomen in.

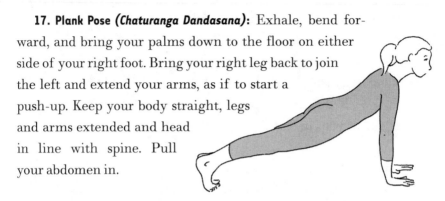

**18. Lowered Plank *(Chatu-ranga Dandasana)*:** Exhale, bending your elbows and lowering your whole body to a few inches off the floor. Draw your elbows back and close to your sides. Then lower yourself to the floor.

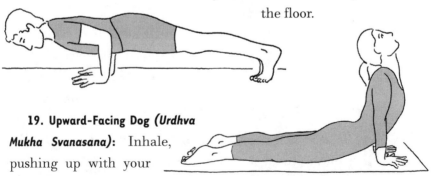

**19. Upward-Facing Dog *(Urdhva Mukha Svanasana)*:** Inhale, pushing up with your arms and chest and arching your back, as in Cobra. Now lift your pelvis and legs slightly off the floor, resting your entire body weight on your hands and the tops of your feet. Draw your torso forward between straight arms and open your chest. Roll your shoulder blades down and keep your buttocks firm to protect your lower back. Abdomen is lifted.

**20. Downward-Facing Dog (*Adho Mukha Svanasana*):** Exhale, lifting your hips up and back as you turn your body into an upside-down V. Keep your arms and legs straight and press your heels to the floor. Shoulders are pressed down and away from the ears.

**21. Chair Pose (*Utkatasana*):** Exhale, walking or jumping your feet forward to between your hands. Inhale as you rise to standing, arms raised toward the ceiling. Exhale as you bend your knees and squat low. Bring your palms together overhead, arms in line with your torso. Pull your abdomen in. Inhale.

**22. Plank Pose (*Chaturanga Dandasana*):** Exhale, bend forward, and place your palms flat on the mat on either side of your feet. Lunge your right leg back, then your left, and extend your arms, as if to start a push-up. Keep your body straight, legs and arms extended and head in line with spine. Pull your abdomen in.

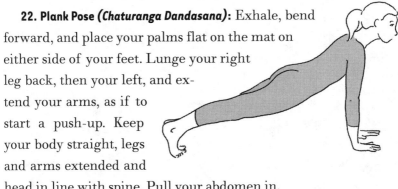

**23. Lowered Plank (*Chaturanga Dandasana*):** Exhale, bending your elbows and lowering your body to a few inches off the floor. Draw your elbows back and close to your sides. Then lower yourself to the floor.

**24. Upward-Facing Dog** *(Urdhva Mukha Svanasana)*: Inhale, pushing up with your arms and chest and arching your back, as in Cobra. Now lift your pelvis and legs slightly off the floor, resting your entire body weight on your hands and the tops of your feet. Draw your torso forward between straight arms and open your chest. Roll your shoulder blades down and keep your buttocks firm to protect your lower back. Abdomen is lifted.

**25. Downward-Facing Dog** *(Adho Mukha Svanasana)*: Exhale, lifting your hips up and back as you turn your body into an upside-down V. Keep your arms and legs straight and press your heels to the floor. Shoulders are pressed down and away from the ears.

**26. Triangle (*Trikonasana*):** Exhale, lunging your right foot forward and turning your left foot out to the side to rest flat. Straighten both legs as you place your right hand on your right shin, and raise your left arm toward the ceiling. Inhale, looking up at your left hand. Pull your abdomen in.

**27. Plank Pose (*Chaturanga Dandasana*):** Exhale, bend forward, and bring your palms down to the floor on either side of your right foot. Bring the right leg back to join the left and extend your arms, as if to start a push-up. Keep your body straight, legs and arms extended and head in line with spine. Pull your abdomen in.

**28. Lowered Plank (*Chaturanga Dandasana*):** Exhale, bending your elbows and lowering your whole body to a few inches off the floor. Draw your elbows back and close to your sides. Then lower yourself to the floor.

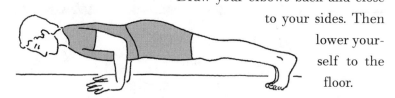

**29. Upward-Facing Dog (*Urdhva Mukha Svanasana*):** Inhale, pushing up with your arms and chest and arching your back, as in Cobra. Now lift your pelvis and legs slightly off the floor, resting your entire body weight on your hands and the tops of your feet. Draw your torso forward between

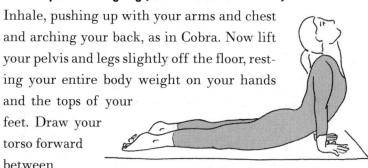

straight arms and open your chest. Roll your shoulder blades down and keep your buttocks firm to protect your lower back. Abdomen is lifted.

**30. Downward-Facing Dog (*Adho Mukha Svanasana*):** Exhale, lifting your hips up and back as you turn your body into an upside-down V. Keep your arms and legs straight and press your heels to the floor. Shoulders are pressed down and away from the ears.

**31. Triangle (*Trikonasana*):** Exhale, lunging your left foot forward and turning your right foot out to the side to rest flat. Straighten both legs as you place your left hand on your left shin, and raise your right arm toward the ceiling. Inhale, looking up at your right hand. Pull your abdomen in.

**32. Mountain Pose (*Tadasana*):** Exhale, lifting your torso upright. Bring your feet together. Bring your palms together over your heart center. Take a few breaths, breathing in light and energy, exhaling tension and fatigue.

## MOON SALUTATION *(CHANDRA NAMASKAR)*

This ancient, classic yoga routine is traditionally done in the evening, to greet and honor the moon. But it can, of course, be practiced at any time of day.

**1. Mountain Pose *(Tadasana)*:** Stand with your feet together, legs straight, kneecaps tightened and pulled up, weight distributed evenly and hands in prayer position over your heart center. Tilt your pelvis under, abdomen pulled in and shoulders relaxed and pulled down, away from your ears. Lift your sternum toward the ceiling.

**2. Standing Side-to-Side *(Nitambasana)*:** Inhale, raising your arms up just behind your ears, your palms facing each other. Think of lifting your arms up and out of your rib cage. Exhale, stretching to the right. Pull your abdomen in. Come to center. Repeat left.

**3. Standing Backbend:** Inhale, come back to center. Tighten your buttock muscles firmly to protect your lower back, lift your sternum toward the ceiling, and arch your spine. Pause for 3 seconds.

**4. Standing Forward Bend (*Uttanasana*):** Exhale, extending your arms forward, and fold forward from the hips, abdomen in. Bend your knees slightly. Relax your face, head, neck, and shoulders toward the floor and lower your chest to your thighs.

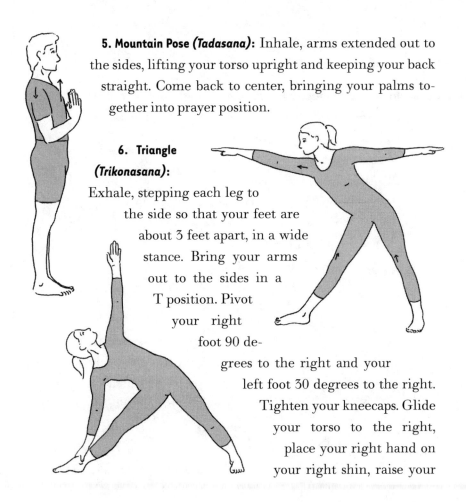

**5. Mountain Pose *(Tadasana)*:** Inhale, arms extended out to the sides, lifting your torso upright and keeping your back straight. Come back to center, bringing your palms together into prayer position.

**6. Triangle *(Trikonasana)*:** Exhale, stepping each leg to the side so that your feet are about 3 feet apart, in a wide stance. Bring your arms out to the sides in a T position. Pivot your right foot 90 degrees to the right and your left foot 30 degrees to the right. Tighten your kneecaps. Glide your torso to the right, place your right hand on your right shin, raise your left arm toward the ceiling, and look up to your left hand. Pull your abdomen in.

**7. Triangle *(Trikonasana)*:** Inhale, straightening your torso and returning your body to center. Exhale; pivot your left foot 90 degrees to the left and your right foot 30 degrees to the left. Tighten your kneecaps. Glide your torso to the left, place your left hand on your left shin, raise your right arm toward the ceiling, and look up to your right hand. Pull your abdomen in.

**8. Side Angle Pose *(Parsvottanasana)*:** Inhale, straighten and return your body to center, then raise your arms above your head. Pivot your right foot 90 degrees to the right, your left foot slightly to the right, and rotate your body to the right to face in the same direction. Tighten your kneecaps. Exhale and bend your torso forward, bringing your forehead to your right knee and placing your hands on either side of your feet.

**9. Side Angle Pose (*Parsvottanasana*):** Inhale, straighten and return your body to center, then raise your arms above your head. Pivot your left foot 90 degrees to the left, your right foot slightly to the left, and rotate your body to the left to face in the same direction. Tighten your kneecaps. Exhale and bend your torso forward, bringing your forehead to your left knee and placing your hands on either side of your feet.

**10. Mountain Pose (*Tadasana*):** Inhale, sweep your arms up above your head, straighten and return to center and bring your feet together. Bring your palms together into prayer position.

If repeating Moon Salutation, proceed directly to Step 2.

# Yoga for Abdominals

## The Abs of Your Dreams

Are you tired of doing an absurd number of crunches to firm your abdominal muscles? You're not alone. One of the questions I field most frequently is, "How can I get rid of the excess weight around my stomach?" The simple answer is yoga practice. By practicing yoga you can create that sleek, sensual stomach you've always dreamed about.

Yoga to improve your abs is easily done at home in just a few minutes a day, without any high-tech equipment. A yoga abs workout will strengthen your stomach muscles and keep you lithe and limber. Practicing yoga to improve your abs will also ease your mind, soothe your soul, and provide you with a new inner sense of balance.

Strong, flexible abdominals not only contribute to an attractive appearance but also perform important physiological functions. Abdominals are your body's core stabilizers for every move you make. They are used for more than holding yoga asanas. Your abdominals are important for breathing, pelvic alignment, torso flexion and rotation, and erect posture, as well as for lumbar spine and digestive organ support. Strong, stable abdominals will improve your posture and assist you in efficiently performing everyday chores, such as picking up your groceries or your children. However, there is a difference between a supple, toned belly and rippled, six-pack abs.

Hollywood, the glamour industry, and the media have conveyed images of flat, taut abs as the epitome of sexiness and beauty. This has created a false standard of an ideal physique. Society's obsession with rock-hard abs has had physical and mental consequences. Doing excessive abdominal crunches and overtraining your abs can lead to chronic stomach-muscle tightness, limited torso flexibility, and muscle imbalance. If the abdominals are inappropriately trained, they become tighter, while the back extensors (the long muscles running parallel to the spine that support and sustain it) become relatively weaker and overstretched. This can lead to a rounded, slumped posture and a weak and vulnerable lower back.

Our culture expects women's bellies to be flat, insidiously rejecting women's sensuality and life-giving power. It exhorts men to display "masculine" vigor with a military posture (sticking their chests out and sucking their stomachs in). In contrast, Eastern practices of yoga, martial arts, and belly dance develop and energize the belly as a source of spiritual, physical, and sensual strength. These practices teach us to listen to our "gut instinct." Yoga emphasizes supple bellies. Practicing yoga will help you develop a perfect balance of abdominal strength and tone. It will also provide a stable core, a center of movement, equanimity, and spiritual power.

## Belly Basics

By requiring you to move and hold your abdominal muscles as a unit, rather than isolate them as you do when you perform crunches, yoga for abs will give you a long, lean look. Yoga exercises all of your abdominal muscles. Holding the postures strengthens the muscles isometrically, toning your abdomen without compromising flexibility. Although traditional crunches also strengthen the abdominals, they require you to collapse into your center. In contrast, yoga poses lengthen your torso, creating a centered and strong feeling and appearance.

The abdominals consist of four sets of muscles—the transversus abdominis, the external obliques, the internal obliques, and the rectus abdominis—that stretch over the internal organs and work in tandem. Your transversus abdominis, the deepest abdominal muscle, runs around your torso horizontally, wrapping it like a corset, and works with the other abdominal muscles to hold in your lower belly. Pranayama, or yoga breathing, is the most effective exercise for the deep transversus. The rectus abdominis (the layer of muscle along the front of the torso and closest to the skin's surface), the external obliques (the muscles found on the sides of the body), and the internal obliques (the muscles found behind the external obliques) are responsible for stabilizing the torso and moving the spine in all directions. The rectus abdominis flexes the trunk and the oblique muscles rotate the trunk.

Holding specific yoga postures will strengthen and tone your stomach muscles. Practicing yoga will also create a dynamic equilibrium between your abs and your lower back by adding strength in a balanced manner. This will strengthen and protect your lower back. It's good to have stomach muscles that are strong. It's equally important to make them flexible with poses, such as Bridge Pose (page 110) and Bow Pose (page 112), that are complementary to the abdominal poses.

By practicing the following abdominal postures at least 3 times a week, you will achieve an overall improvement in the outer appearance of the abdominals. However, don't expect to completely melt away belly fat by just performing these yoga asanas. It's not realistic to spot-reduce this or any other area of your body. To lose excess fat, and reach and maintain your perfect weight, combine these asanas with a healthy diet and a Yoga Power Workout from Chapter 3, as shown in the Maintenance Yoga Power and Abdominals Workout Plan that follows (page 97).

## The 10-Minute Yoga for Abs Workout

If your time is limited, yoga abdominal poses can be practiced on their own. You will reap benefits even if you have only 10 minutes a day to do this yoga practice. If you have more time, combine this 10-minute workout with any of the Yoga Power Workouts in Chapter 3. For example, see the combination Maintenance Yoga Power and Abdominals Workout that follows.

Be aware that it may take you more than 4 weeks to do this routine comfortably, depending on your physical condition. If you feel comfortable and confident doing the poses in Weeks 1 and 2, proceed to Weeks 3 and 4. Otherwise, stay with Weeks 1 and 2 until you feel strong enough to continue.

## Weeks 1 and 2

**Workout Schedule:** Practice for 10 minutes, 3 times a week.

**Yoga Abdominals:** For each workout, perform at least 2 of the first 6 poses and finish with Bridge Pose and Complete Breath.

### Choose two:
Half Boat Pose
Modified Revolved Abdomen Pose
Revolved Abdomen Pose
Single Leg Lifts
Seated Forward Bend
Stomach Lift

### Plus:
Bridge Pose
Complete Breath

## Weeks 3 and 4

**Workout Schedule:** Practice for 10 minutes, 3 times a week.

**Yoga Abdominals:** For each workout, perform at least 2 of the first 6 poses and finish with Bow Pose and Breath of Fire.

**Choose two:**

Half Boat Pose

Boat Pose

Boat Pose Variation

Revolved Abdomen Pose

Double Leg Lifts

Seated Forward Bend

Lowered Plank

**Plus:**

Bow Pose

Breath of Fire

## Maintenance Yoga Power and Abdominals Workout Plan

A combination of the 10-Minute Yoga for Abs and the Maintenance Yoga Power Workout will help you to build and maintain your strength, cardiovascular fitness, and flexibility.

## Weeks 1 and Beyond

**Workout Schedule:** Alternate Sun Salutations A, B, C, and D and Moon Salutation practice 5 days a week for 20 minutes. On practice days 1, 3, and 5, follow your Sun Salutation practice with 10 minutes of Yoga Abdominals poses. Finish all five workouts with 20 minutes of your favorite aerobic activity, such as walking, easy jogging, treadmill walking/jogging, or stationary cycling, 4 or 5 days a week for 20 minutes.

**Warm Up:** Perform Sun Salutation A once slowly, holding each posture for 5 breaths.

**Sun Salutation:** Perform 4 to 6 repetitions of Sun Salutation A, B, or C, or 1 Sun Salutation D and 1 Moon Salutation, with increasing speed, holding each pose for 1 to 3 breaths. Pace yourself at 50 to 65 percent of your maximum heart rate.

**Yoga for Abs:** 10 minutes of Yoga for Abs Workout.

**Aerobics:** 20 minutes of aerobic activity plus three intervals, 1 minute each, of higher-intensity activity. For example, if you're walking, walk 5 minutes, then speed-walk or do an easy jog for 1 minute; repeat the sequence 2 times. Continue walking for the remainder of the time. If you're jogging, then sprint during the 1-minute intervals; if you're stationary cycling, add 1-minute intervals of jumping rope; if you're treadmill walking, increase your speed or incline. Pace yourself at 50 to 65 percent of your maximum heart rate.

**Cool Down:** Perform Sun Salutation A once slowly, holding each posture for 5 breaths. End with 5 to 10 minutes of Supported Relaxation Pose (page 168).

## Asanas for Abs

## HALF BOAT POSE *(MODIFIED NAVASANA)*

**What It Does:** It tones and strengthens your rectus abdominis muscle. This is a simpler version of the traditional Boat Pose. You can still reap benefits by doing this beginner's posture.

**How to Do It:**

1. Sit on the floor with your knees bent in front of you hip-width apart and feet flat on the floor. With your hands, hold the backs of your thighs, close to your knees.

2. Lean back, lift your legs so your calves are parallel to the floor, and balance on your sit bones.

3. Inhale, then exhale. Now straighten your arms forward, parallel to the floor, palms facing each other. If this is too difficult, hold the backs of your thighs with your hands. Draw your navel back toward your spine. Work up to holding this pose for 30 seconds. Balance and breathe!

4. Exhale and bring your feet to the floor.

5. Repeat 3 times.

## BOAT POSE AND BOAT POSE VARIATION
### (NAVASANA AND NAVASANA VARIATION)

**What It Does:** It tones and strengthens the rectus abdominis muscle. This is an intermediate-level posture, more advanced than the Half Boat Pose. Individuals with back injuries should not practice this without the assistance of an experienced teacher.

**How to Do It:**

1. Sit on the floor with your knees bent in front of you hip-width apart and feet flat on the floor. With your hands hold the backs of your thighs, close to your knees.

2. Lean back, lift your feet so your calves are parallel to the floor, and balance on your sit bones.

3. Inhale; then exhale, extending your legs until they are straight, balancing in a V position. Straighten your arms forward, parallel to the floor, palms facing each other. Draw your navel back toward your spine. Use your abdominals to stay balanced and lifted, elongating your spine. Work up to holding this pose for 30 seconds. Balance and breathe!

4. Exhale and bring your feet to the floor.

5. Repeat 3 times.

6. As you get stronger, add this variation to your practice: Go into the Boat Pose, then slowly lower your legs and arms until they're both just an inch or so off

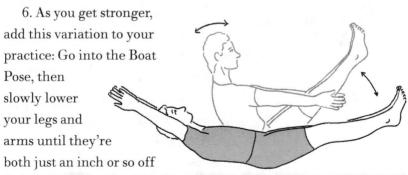

the mat. Pause. Don't strain! Smoothly bring arms and legs back up to Boat Pose. Build up to 3 repetitions.

## MODIFIED REVOLVED ABDOMEN POSE
### (MODIFIED JATHARA PARIVARTANASANA)

**What It Does:** It exercises the external and internal obliques and strengthens the abdominal wall. This is a simpler version of the Revolved Abdomen Pose. You can still reap benefits by doing this beginner's posture.

**How to Do It:**

1. Lie on your back, knees pulled in toward your chest. Keep your lower back in contact with the floor. Straighten your arms out to the sides in a T position at shoulder level, palms down.

2. Exhale; keeping your knees together, slowly lower them to the right

while keeping your shoulders in contact with the floor. Touch the floor with the outside of your right foot. Gaze toward your left hand.

3. Relax for 3 full breaths.

4. Inhale; then use your abs and raise your knees back to starting position.

5. Repeat on the left side.

6. Repeat for 2 more cycles.

## REVOLVED ABDOMEN POSE (JATHARA PARIVARTANASANA)

**What It Does:** It exercises the external and internal obliques and strengthens the abdominal wall. This is an intermediate-level posture.

**How to Do It:**

1. Lie on your back, knees pulled in to your chest. Keep your lower back in contact with the floor. Straighten your arms out to the sides in a T position at shoulder level, your palms down.

2. Inhale, straightening your legs to vertical and forming a 90-degree angle. Keep your feet together and hold this leg-trunk position throughout the asana.

3. Exhale; using your abs to control the momentum, slowly lower your legs toward the right side while keeping your shoulders in contact with the floor. Touch the floor with the outside of your right foot. Gaze toward your left hand.

4. Relax for 3 full breaths.

5. Inhale; then use your abs to raise your legs back to vertical.

6. Repeat on the left side.

7. Repeat for 3 more cycles.

## SINGLE LEG LIFT
### (MODIFIED URDHAVA PRASARITA PADASANA)

**What It Does:** It strengthens your entire abdomen, especially the lower rectus abdominis, and the lower back. It also increases your stamina. This is a simpler version of the Double Leg Lift. You can still reap benefits with this beginner's posture.

### How to Do It:

1. Lie on your back with knees bent and feet flat on the floor. Arms extend out to the sides, palms are down.

2. Inhale, straightening your right leg to vertical and forming a 90-degree angle. Extend your heel.

4. Exhale. Using your abdominals, tilt your pelvis under, keeping your lower back flat to the floor, and slowly lower your right leg. If you have difficulty maintaining the pelvic tilt and keeping your lower back flat in contact with the floor, slip your hands under your buttocks, thumbs touching. As you progress, check periodically to see if you're strong enough to do this pose without the extra support.

5. Repeat 3 times on the right, inhaling as your leg goes up, exhaling as your leg goes down.

6. Repeat Steps 1 through 5 with left leg.

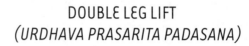

## DOUBLE LEG LIFT
### *(URDHAVA PRASARITA PADASANA)*

**What It Does:** It strengthens your entire abdomen, especially the lower rectus abdominis, and the lower back. It also significantly increases your stamina. Do not do this posture if you have lower-back problems. This is an intermediate-advanced posture and should be attempted only when the Single Leg Lift has been mastered.

**How to Do It:**

1. Lie on your back, both legs extended, arms at your sides, palms down.

2. Draw your knees to your chest.

3. Inhale, straightening your legs to vertical. Keep your feet together and flex your heels.

4. Exhale as you use your abdominals to tilt your pelvis under and keep your lumbar spine flat to the floor. Now lower your legs to a

60-degree angle. Hold for 10 seconds, concentrating on lengthening the abdominal muscles.

5. Lower your legs to 30 degrees and pause for another 10 seconds.

6. Lower your legs to 4 inches off the floor and hold for 10 seconds.

7. Inhale; then exhale, bringing both legs up toward the ceiling.

8. Rest; then repeat.

## SEATED FORWARD BEND
### (PASCHIMOTTANASANA)

**What It Does:** It tones the abdominal wall and organs, especially the upper rectus abdominis muscle, calms the nerves, and quiets the mind. Do not do this posture if you have lower-back problems.

**How to Do It:**

1. Sit with your legs stretched out in front of you. Reach down, place your hands under your thighs, and pull the thigh muscles out to the sides.

2. With legs extended, inhale and raise your arms up toward the ceiling, your palms facing each other.

3. Exhale, keeping your neck relaxed and your spine elongated, and smoothly extending your body forward. Lead with the breastbone.

4. Inhale and extend the body forward a bit further. Grasp your calves, ankles, or feet. Try to keep your back straight. Knees are straight. Draw your abdominal muscles upward to extend the forward bend.

5. If your back rounds excessively or you cannot extend forward enough to hold your calves, ankles, or feet, loop a towel or strap around the bottom of your feet and use the ends to help you extend your torso forward. Hold this pose for 30 seconds.

6. If you're ready, deepen the pose by continuing the forward motion. If you've already reached your edge, hold where you are. Do not force this pose! Flexibility will come with further practice.

7. If you are able, continue the forward motion, with feet flexed, toes pulled back. Rest your abdomen, chest, and head on your legs. Your elbows and forearms now rest on the floor, palms down.

8. Maintain a steady focus on your breathing, playing the edge of

your stretch. Inhale and pull back, relaxing; then exhale and stretch forward right to your edge.

9. Hold for 30 seconds, working up to as long as you wish.

## PLANK POSE AND LOWERED PLANK
### (CHATURANGA DANDASANA)

**What It Does:** It creates a strong and balanced body. All of the abdominals work together to hold this pose.

**How to Do It:**

1. Lie on your stomach with your hands flat on the floor under your shoulders (think push-up position). The toes are curled under.

2. Push yourself up until your arms are straight (don't lock the elbows), keeping shoulders pulled back and down. Draw 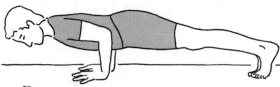 your navel in toward your spine and allow your abs to support your body as you hold the pose for 30 seconds.

3. If you have difficulty holding this pose, do not continue. Simply lower yourself to the floor.

4. If you can hold this Plank Pose, try bending your elbows and lowering your entire body toward the floor. Lower as far as you can (but not all the way!) without rounding your shoulders forward, lifting your buttocks up, or letting your hips sag. Use your abdominals to hold the pose. Try to maintain equal body weight between your hands and feet. Ideally, hold for 30 seconds. Breathe!

5. Lower your body to the floor.

6. Repeat. Build up to 5 repetitions.

## COMPLEMENTARY ASANAS

Complete your abdominal work with the following asanas that stretch your abdominal muscles, to develop a perfect balance of abdominal strength, tone, and suppleness.

## BRIDGE POSE *(SETU BANDHASANA)*

**What It Does:** It stretches the abdominal muscles, increases flexibility in the spine, and firms the buttocks.

**How to Do It:**

1. Lie on your back, arms along your sides, your palms down. Bend both knees and place your feet flat on the floor, hip distance apart.

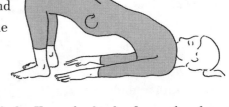

2. Tilt your pelvis, pressing the small of your back gently to the floor. Inhale. Keep the back of your head on the floor. Exhale slowly as you raise your hips up to the middle of the shoulders one vertebra at a time, using your abdominals (building a bridge). Stabilize by pressing down on your heels. Tighten your buttocks and tilt your pelvis under. Hold for 6 seconds.

3. Exhale slowly as you lower your back to the floor, one vertebra at a time.

4. Repeat 3 times.

## BOW POSE
## (DHANURASANA)

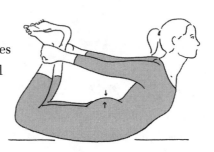

**What It Does:** It stretches and tones the abdominal muscles, increases flexibility in the spine, increases stamina, and firms the buttocks.

**How to Do It:**

1. Lie on your stomach with your forehead on the mat. Reach back and grasp your ankles firmly, keeping your knees hip-distance apart. Arms are straight.

2. Inhale, then exhale, lifting your forehead, nose, and chin. Raise your chest off the floor. To protect your lower back, tighten your buttocks and tuck your pelvis under. Raise your knees off the floor.

3. Inhale, squeeze your shoulder blades together, and lift your breastbone up. Relax your neck.

4. Exhale, releasing the intensity of the stretch slightly, then inhale, lifting your chest and rib cage a little further.

5. Hold for a moment. Exhale and release the stretch slightly, then inhale and lift the chest even higher.

6. Release hands from ankles and lie on your stomach. Rest for a moment.

7. Repeat 2 times.

## BELLY BREATHING

According to yoga philosophy, prana is life force energy. Pranayama breathing is the conscious regulation of the breath that circulates revitalizing prana throughout the body. Pranayama practice exercises all the muscles of the abdomen, firming and toning your stomach.

## COMPLETE BREATH (*PRANAYAMA*)

**What It Does:** Research indicates that breathing slowly and deeply sends a message to the body and mind that all is well, thereby interrupting the stress cycle. Deep, diaphragmatic breathing requires all of the abdominal muscles to compress and expel the air from the lungs completely.

**How to Do It:**

1. Sit comfortably in a chair, or on the floor in a cross-legged position. Keep your back straight and your neck and head aligned with your spinal column.

2. Breathe in slowly through your nose (mouth closed!) to the count of 4. Allow your diaphragm to descend, expanding the middle rib cage, then expanding the base of the lungs. Hold for a moment.

3. Breathe out through the nose, releasing the air slowly to the count of 8. Exhale from the upper lobes of the lungs, then the middle rib cage. Slightly contract your abdominal muscles and squeeze all the air out.

4. Repeat 6 times.

## STOMACH LIFT (*UDDIYANA BANDHA*)

**What It Does:** It strengthens the abdominal muscles and keeps them flexible; tones and massages the abdominal organs and glands. Practice on an empty stomach.

**How to Do It:**

1. Stand with your feet hip-distance apart. Bend forward with your knees bent. Place your hands on

your thighs above the knees for leverage. Lean the weight of your torso into your hands.

2. Exhale forcefully from your mouth. Close your mouth and bring your chin to your throat. Hold the exhalation and pull your abdomen back toward the spine and up toward the solar plexus.

3. Hold for 2 seconds, then rhythmically pump the abdominal muscles in and out with a pull-in, release motion, 5 or more times.

4. Before the lack of oxygen becomes uncomfortable, relax the abdominals and inhale slowly. Stand up.

## BREATH OF FIRE, OR BELLOWS BREATH
### *(BHASTRIKA PRANAYAMA)*

**What It Does:** These forceful exhalations provide a good workout for the transversus abdominis muscle. Like a bellows, which draws in air and blows it across heated coals to create more heat, bhastrika generates more heat and circulation in the body. Practice bhastrika daily on an empty stomach. Bhastrika increases intra-abdominal pressure and should not be practiced by individuals with heart disease, high blood pressure, or digestive disorders, or by women during menstruation or pregnancy.

**How to Do It:**

1. Sit comfortably in a cross-legged position on the floor. Pull your navel in as you exhale deeply and sharply through pursed lips. Breathe quickly through your nose by forcing air out with sharp, deep, pulling-in movements at the navel. The inhalation is a response to the exhalation.

2. Do 10 exhalations at the rate of 1 breath per second. If the strength of your exhalation begins to weaken, reduce the number of breaths. Build up to 3 rounds of 10 breaths each, and rest as needed between rounds.

3. As you grow stronger, gradually increase to 2 breaths per second and 20 exhalations per round. Repeat up to 3 rounds.

# chapter 5

# Yoga for Toning

## Get Toned, Lean, and Fit

A yoga workout has the power to tone you from head to toe, help you lose fat, teach you good posture, build muscle, and reduce the appearance of cellulite. Because yoga emphasizes strengthening and stretching equally, it is an ideal way to tone your body while improving your flexibility. Since yoga combines strength training with intense stretching, practicing it will help you develop muscles that are strong, lean, and long. This will help you look thinner, taller, and healthier.

When you lose muscle tone, the skin that supports the muscles of your butt, hips, thighs, and arms sags. For a firm body, taut skin, and maintenance of muscle tone, you'll need to strengthen those muscles. Although you can't spot-reduce, you can tighten flabby areas with these muscle-targeted yoga postures.

Over the years, I've found that combining the Yoga Power Workouts from Chapter 3 with supersculpting asanas maximizes every workout. The Yoga Power routines burn overall body fat, while strength training asanas tone and define those out-of-shape areas.

Toned muscles not only are essential for a healthy physique, but also play an important role in a weight management program. Toned, strong muscles supercharge your metabolism, helping you to burn additional calories during the day so you can reach and maintain your ideal weight. Toned muscles also give you improved posture and overall appearance. You'll use your muscles more efficiently, avoid injuries, and boost endurance.

## Supersculpting Yoga

Yoga is widely hailed as a great way to improve flexibility, balance, and relaxation. But what's not as well known is that yoga can build muscles. Yoga postures have been developed to efficiently stretch every muscle in your body slowly and gently as a type of moving meditation. Holding yoga poses in this way develops what's called isometric strength. Yoga poses use the body's own weight to provide resistance against gravity, and this results in strong, lean, and limber muscles. You'll become toned and strong but never bulky, because you're working through a full range of motion using your own body weight as resistance.

Yoga builds muscle endurance rather than the pure power you develop from weight lifting. As you practice the asanas that follow, focus on maintaining proper body alignment while activating the appropriate muscles and breathing deeply.

## Strength Training

Although supersculpting asanas can make you strong and toned, I've found that the addition of free weights to a yoga practice can be very useful. Yoga postures with free weights improve dynamic strength: your muscles become shorter and thicker, protecting you against loss of bone and muscle mass.

Ultimately, doing yoga poses without weights will not build as much muscle mass as training with weights. Without weights, the maximum load you carry is limited to your body weight. This may be an issue if you're an intermediate or advanced yoga practitioner. If your muscles have adapted to supporting your body weight, then your regular routine no longer presents a rigorous strength-building, toning challenge. Working with weights can help the more advanced practitioner gain greater strength, stability, and stamina.

Weights are also beneficial for beginners who have trouble supporting their body weight in asanas such as Plank Pose or Crow Pose. Training with weights can help beginners build the strength and stamina necessary to support their own body weight in yoga poses.

It's best to begin with light weights. I generally recommend that beginners start with 1-pound weights. As with any exercise program, start slowly and build up gradually. Always move your weight through the largest range of motion possible, but don't hyperextend joints. As you advance, increase the weight to fatigue your target muscles by the end of each set.

Yoga toning asanas with and without weights will build more than just the muscles. The mental focus required to hold a yoga pose also builds equanimity, along with mental and spiritual clarity.

## Perfect Yoga Posture

Good posture instantly makes you look toned, taller, and thinner. Yoga teaches beautiful posture and the basics of body alignment, since most poses require a conscious lengthening of the spine, a lifted chest, shoulders that are held back, and firm abdominals. Good posture improves more than just aesthetics; it substantially reduces the risk of pain and injury, especially in the lower back.

Slouching is often caused by an imbalance of opposing muscle groups. People with poor posture typically have tight hamstrings, tight chest muscles, weak abdominals, and weak upper-back muscles. This causes rounded shoulders and a hunched-over look, protruding abdominals, and sagging buttocks. The following supersculpting asanas will focus on toning, stretching, and strengthening muscles in these areas, to help get rid of that slouch.

## Anticellulite Yoga Toning

If you have cellulite, or want to prevent its appearance, this Yoga Toning Workout is for you. The key to banishing cellulite is to lose the fat and build muscle. The more taut your skin is, the less cellulite will show. By combining Yoga Power Workouts from Chapter 3 to burn overall body fat (or cellulite) with Yoga Toning to strengthen key muscles, you can produce major reductions in the appearance of cellulite.

Cellulite is fat, like any other fat. The only difference is the way the fat is deposited under the skin. Pockets of this fat will cause the overlying skin to dimple, creating a lumpy appearance on the hips, buttocks, and thighs. Cellulite appears in men and women, although it's more common in women because they have a higher percentage of fat on their bodies. The size and thickness of cellulite are also genetically determined and age-related.

Miracle thigh creams, starving, yoga, and even surgery won't guarantee permanent removal of stubborn cellulite. However, a combination of Yoga Power Workouts, supersculpting asanas, and a balanced, low-fat diet, as described in Chapter 7, will reduce or prevent the appearance of cellulite.

## Yoga Toning Practice Plan

Are you ready to make your yoga practice do more for you? It's as easy as adding a few supersculpting asanas to your Yoga Power Workout. In just a few weeks, you'll be slimmer, stronger, and more toned.

If your time is limited, supersculpting asanas can be practiced on their own. You will reap benefits even if you have only 10 minutes a day to do this yoga practice. If you have more time, you can incorporate this 10-minute workout into any of the Yoga Power Workouts in Chapter 3 (see the Maintenance Yoga Power and Toning Workout that follows). To burn additional calories and achieve an even more efficient workout, add Yoga for Abdominals (see Chapter 4) to your Yoga Power and Toning Workout on alternate days.

Be aware that it may take you more than 4 weeks to do this routine comfortably, depending on your physical condition. If you feel comfortable and confident doing the poses in Weeks 1 and 2, proceed to Weeks 3 and 4. Otherwise, stay with Weeks 1 and 2 until you feel strong enough to continue.

## Weeks 1 and 2

**Workout Schedule:** Practice for 10 minutes, 2 or 3 days per week, taking a day off between training sessions.

### Supersculpting Asanas—Choose at Least 2:
Half Shoulderstand/Fish Pose
Cow's-Head Pose
Dolphin Headstand Preparation
Salute to Gods and Goddesses

Inclined Plane

Locust Pose

## Weeks 3 and 4

**Workout Schedule:** Practice for 10 minutes, 2 or 3 days per week, taking a day off between training sessions.

**Supersculpting Asanas—Choose 2:**

Revolved Triangle Pose

Extended Hand-to-Big-Toe Pose

Bound Lunge

Crow Pose

Locust Pose with Leg Weights

Chair Pose with Weights

Side Bend with Weights

## Maintenance Yoga Power and Toning Workout

A combination of Yoga Toning Practice and the Maintenance Yoga Power Workout will help you build and maintain your strength, cardiovascular fitness, and flexibility.

## Week 1 and Beyond

**Workout Schedule:** Alternate Sun Salutations A, B, C, and D and Moon Salutation practice 5 days a week for 20 minutes. On practice days 1, 3, and 5, follow with 10 minutes of Yoga Toning Practice. Finish each of these workouts with 20 minutes of your favorite aerobic activity, such as walking, easy jogging, treadmill walking/jogging, or stationary cycling.

**Warm Up:** Perform Sun Salutation A once slowly, holding each posture for 5 breaths.

**Sun Salutation:** Perform 4 to 6 repetitions of Sun Salutation A, B, or C, or 1 Sun Salutation D and 1 Moon Salutation, with increasing speed, holding each pose for 1 to 3 breaths. Pace yourself at 50 to 65 percent of your maximum heart rate.

**Yoga Toning:** 10 minutes of Yoga Toning Practice.

**Aerobics:** 20 minutes of aerobic activity plus 3 intervals, 1 minute each, of higher-intensity activity. For example, if you're walking, walk 5 minutes, then speed-walk or do an easy jog for 1 minute; repeat the sequence 2 times. Continue walking for the remainder of the time. If you're jogging, then sprint for 1-minute intervals; if you're stationary cycling, add 1 minute intervals of jumping rope; if you're treadmill walking, increase your speed or incline. Pace yourself at 50 to 65 percent of your maximum heart rate.

**Cool Down:** Perform 1 repetition of Sun Salutation A slowly, holding each posture for 5 breaths. End with 5 to 10 minutes of Supported Relaxation Pose (page 168).

## Supersculpting Asanas

By practicing these supersculpting yoga postures you can get toned, lean, and fit.

## HALF SHOULDERSTAND (ARDHA SARVANGASANA)

**What It Does:** This classic posture tones and strengthens the entire body. This is a simpler version of and preparation for the full shoulderstand, which requires the supervision of a qualified instructor. To protect your neck, practice on a neatly folded towel or blanket, with your shoulders 3 to 4 inches from the folded edge and your head on the mat. You can still reap full shoulderstand benefits by doing this beginner's posture. Always follow with Fish Pose.

**How to do It:**

1. Lie on your back, feet together, hands at your sides. Inhale, raising straight legs toward the ceiling.

2. Exhale and raise your hips off the floor, using your hands to push off. Support your pelvis with your hands cupped around your hips, elbows close together. Keep your legs at a 45-degree angle.

3. Hold the pose for 30 to 60 seconds. Breathe comfortably.

4. Bend both knees to your forehead; bring your hands to the floor. Slowly and with control, bring your hips to the floor. Straighten your legs and lower them to the floor. If your back and abdominal muscles are weak, bend your knees to your forehead and lower your bent legs to the floor.

## FISH POSE (MATSYASANA)

**What It Does:** Always do Fish Pose after Half Shoulderstand.

It opens the neck and throat, thereby stimulating the thyroid area. This circulation of fresh blood is believed to improve the metabolism, helping you reach or maintain your ideal weight naturally.

**How to Do It:**

1. Lie on your back, legs extended, thighs touching. Slide your hands, palms down, under your buttocks.

2. Inhale, arch your back, and lift your chest away from the floor, placing your weight on your elbows. Squeeze your shoulder blades together. Roll your head back and lightly touch the floor with the crown of your head.

3. Build up to 2 breaths while holding the position. If your neck feels painful or weak, immediately come out of the position.

## COW'S-HEAD POSE (*GOMUKHASANA*)

**What It Does:** It improves posture by developing flexibility in the chest, shoulders, upper back, hips, and legs.

**How to Do It:**

1. Begin seated, with legs extended in front of you. Cross your bent right knee over your left leg so that your right foot rests beside your left hip. Rocking back on your sit bones, bend your left leg so that your left foot rests beside your right hip. Now raise your right arm overhead and reach behind you as if to scratch your back. Reach your left arm behind your back, hand pointing up. Clasp your hands firmly between your shoulder blades. (If you can't clasp hands, hold the end of a towel or strap with your 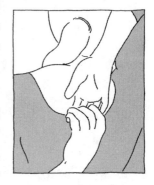 left hand and grab the other end with your right hand. Gradually work your hands closer together on the towel.)

2. Keep your head erect, feel the stretch, and hold the pose for 3 slow, deep breaths.

3. Unclasp your hands, straighten your legs, and repeat on the other side.

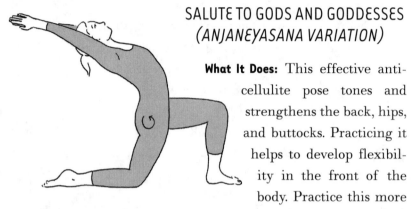

## SALUTE TO GODS AND GODDESSES
### (ANJANEYASANA VARIATION)

**What It Does:** This effective anti-cellulite pose tones and strengthens the back, hips, and buttocks. Practicing it helps to develop flexibility in the front of the body. Practice this more advanced posture when you feel comfortable and strong doing Lunges (page 56).

**How to Do It:**

1. From a kneeling position, bring your left leg forward, placing your left foot flat on the floor. Place your hands on your left knee, maintaining balance.

2. Bring your arms overhead, your palms together, thumbs crossed. Inhale, lift, and bend backward, tightening your buttock muscles firmly and tilting your pelvis under, to protect your lower back. Look up. Hold for 10 seconds.

3. Slowly come up to starting position, contracting your abdominals. Place your hands on your left knee, maintaining balance.

4. Repeat on the other side.

### REVOLVED TRIANGLE POSE (PARIVARTTA TRIKONASANA)

**What It Does:** Revolved Triangle is a combination of a forward bend, a twist, and a balancing pose. It tones and strengthens the legs and buttocks, develops flexibility in the hips and lower back, and trims the waistline. Practice this more advanced posture when you feel comfortable and strong doing Triangle (page 82) and Standing Forward Bend (page 56). Individuals with disc injuries should not practice this or other twisting poses without the assistance of an experienced teacher.

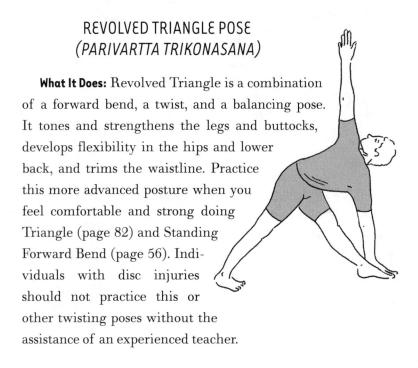

**How to Do It:**

1. Assume a wide stance, feet 3 to 4 feet apart, arms out to the sides in a T position. Pivot your left foot 90 degrees to the left and your right foot 30 degrees to the left, so that your left heel is in line with the arch of your right foot. Square your hips to face your left foot.

2. Exhale, rotating your torso and bending forward, and resting the fingertips of your right hand on the outside of your left foot. Stretch your left arm overhead. Pull your abdomen in. If it is comfortable to do so, turn your head to look up. (If you can't reach the floor, rest your right hand on a chair or block.)

3. Keep reaching, lifting, and lengthening as you hold the pose for 3 or 4 breaths.

4. Straighten up and repeat on the other side.

# BOUND LUNGE *(ANJANEYASANA VARIATION)*

**What It Does:** This effective anticellulite standing lunge tones and strengthens the legs and buttocks. It improves posture by developing flexibility in the chest and shoulders. Practice this more advanced posture when you feel comfortable and strong doing Raised Runner (page 73) and Chest Expander (page 29).

**How to Do It:**

1. From standing, step your right foot straight back, with the ball of the foot pressing into the floor. Place your hands on your left knee, maintaining balance.

2. When ready, clasp your hands behind your back and gently squeeze your shoulder blades together. Straighten your elbows and tighten your buttocks. Inhale, expanding your chest and lifting your arms and chin. Exhale, bringing your hands forward to rest on your left knee.

3. Repeat on the other side.

# EXTENDED-HAND-TO-BIG-TOE POSE
## (UTTHITA HASTA PADANGUSTHASANA)

**What It Does:** This intense, overall body toner strengthens the legs and buttocks as it stretches the hips and hamstrings. It also improves posture by developing superb balance. Practice this more advanced posture when you feel comfortable and strong doing Seated Forward Bend (page 107). Hold on to a wall or chair at first, if you find yourself losing your balance.

**How to Do It:**

1. Begin in Mountain Pose (page 27). Raise your right knee and grab the big toe of your right foot with your right hand. Place your left hand on your left hip and inhale, maintaining balance on your left leg.

2. Exhale and extend the right leg out in front of you, as much as you can. Press your shoulders down and away from your ears. Stretch and balance for 2 or 3 breaths.

3. If you're unable to straighten your right leg, place a strap or

towel around the ball of your right foot and hold the ends with your right hand. Stretch and balance for 2 or 3 breaths.

4. Repeat on the other side.

## DOLPHIN HEADSTAND PREPARATION (ARDHA SIRSANA)

**What It Does:** This tones and strengthens the entire body, especially the arms, shoulders, and neck. Dolphin is a preparation for the headstand, which requires the supervision of a qualified instructor. Practice this on a mat with a neatly folded blanket or padding for your head. You can still reap headstand benefits by doing this preparation.

**How to Do It:**

1. Kneel on a mat and then rest your forearms in front of you on the mat, so that your thighs and upper arms are perpendicular to the floor. Measure the distance between your elbows by placing your left fist against your right elbow. Elbows should be shoulder-width apart.

Interlace your fingers, forming a triangular base with your forearms. Place the crown of your head on the floor, supporting it with cupped hands.

2. Exhale and lift your hips, straightening your knees, with the balls of your feet pressing into the mat. Press your upper arms and

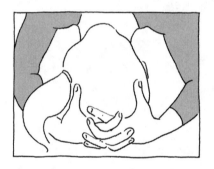

the center of your forearms (the ulna) into the mat to create leverage. Draw your shoulders away from your neck. The top of each wrist is directly over the bottom of the wrist, not tilting in or out.

3. Inhale, push down on your forearms, and lift your head a few inches off the floor. Exhale and bring the crown of your head back down to the mat. Repeat 3 times.

4. Bend your knees and lower them to the mat. Keep your head down for a few moments before sitting up.

# INCLINED PLANE (*PURVOTTANASANA*)

**What It Does:** This powerful posture tones and strengthens the entire body, especially the chest, arms, wrists, shoulders, and buttocks.

**How to Do It:**

1. Sit on the floor with your legs extended in front of you. Place your palms on the floor 6 to 12 inches behind your hips, fingers pointing away from your feet. (If this is difficult, place your hands with fingers pointing toward your feet.) Inhale and squeeze your shoulder blades together.

2. Exhale and lift your hips off the floor. Straighten your arms and legs. Tighten your buttocks, squeeze your shoulder blades together, and extend your chest. Push your heels into the floor. Stretch your neck back as far as possible without discomfort. Breathe and hold, building up to 30 seconds. Keep lifting the hips up.

3. Exhale and lower yourself to the floor.

# CROW POSE (KAKASANA)

**What It Does:** This intense, overall body toner strengthens the arms, chest, and thighs and stretches the hips and back. It also improves posture by developing superb balance. Practice this more advanced posture when you feel comfortable and strong doing Plank Pose and modified Plank Pose (page 57). This is a challenging pose, but as you practice it you will find your balance in the posture.

**How to Do It:**

1. Squat down, resting your weight on the balls of your feet. Place your hands on the floor between your legs, with fingers spread wide. Bring your knees onto the back of your arms (your triceps). Shift your weight forward onto your arms as you rise up on your toes. Press your shoulder blades down and squeeze your inner thighs together.

2. Continue shifting your weight forward, lifting your toes off the floor and slowly balancing yourself. All your weight is resting on your hands.

3. Breathe evenly as you stay balanced and focused. Hold for 30 seconds.

## LOCUST POSE (SALABHASANA)

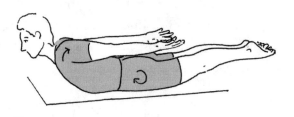

**What It Does:** This is an excellent anti-cellulite toner and strengthener for buttocks, hamstrings, and back. It will also improve posture by reducing rounding of the upper back. Individuals with back problems should not practice full Locust without the assistance of an experienced teacher. You may want to practice this on a mat with a neatly folded blanket or some padding underneath your chest, abdomen, and hips.

**How to Do It:**

1. Lie face down on the mat with your arms stretched down along your sides, your palms up and your forehead on the floor.

2. Inhale, lifting your chest, head, and right leg off the floor. To protect your lower back, pull your abdomen in and tuck your pelvis

under, tighten your buttocks, and keep both hips firmly on the mat. Hold for 3 seconds.

3. Exhale, lowering your chest, head, and leg together slowly to the floor.

4. Repeat Steps 2 and 3 with your left leg.

5. Repeat Steps 2 and 3, this time raising both legs off the floor, along with both arms. This is the full Locust Pose.

6. Release, lie flat, and relax.

## LOCUST POSE WITH LEG WEIGHTS
### (SALABHASANA VARIATION)

**What It Does:** Using leg weights will supercharge lower-body toning and strengthening. Practice this after you've come to feel comfortable and strong when doing the full Locust Pose. Individuals with back problems should not practice this pose.

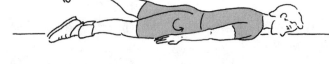

**How to Do It:**

1. Wearing ankle weights that are appropriate for you, lie face down on the mat with arms stretched down along your sides, palms down, and chin on the floor. I recommend 1-pound weights to start.

2. Slowly and with control, inhale and raise your right leg, keeping the leg straight. To protect your lower back, pull your abdomen in and tuck your pelvis under, tighten buttocks, and keep both hips firmly on the mat.

3. Slowly and with control, exhale as you lower your leg to the floor.

4. Repeat with your left leg.

5. Repeat 3 times on each side. Release and relax.

## CHAIR POSE WITH WEIGHTS
### (UTKATASANA VARIATION)

**What It Does:** The use of weights while doing Chair Pose will supercharge lower-body toning and strengthening. Practice this after you've come to feel comfortable and strong when doing Chair Pose.

**How to Do It:**

1. Holding light dumbells that are appropriate for you, stand with your feet hip-width apart. I recommend 1-pound weights to start.

2. Inhale, bend your knees, and squat slowly. Pull your abdomen in and hold your torso erect. Knees are in line with feet. Squat, bringing your thighs as close to horizontal as possible.

3. Exhale, slowly rising to standing.

4. Repeat 3 times.

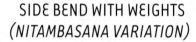

## SIDE BEND WITH WEIGHTS
### (*NITAMBASANA VARIATION*)

**What It Does:** The use of weights while doing Side Bends will supercharge upper-body toning and strengthening and trim the waistline. Practice this after you've come to feel comfortable and strong when doing the Side Bend.

**How to Do It:**

1. Holding two dumbbells that are appropriate for you, inhale and raise your arms straight overhead. Palms face each other and

arms lift up out of the rib cage. I recommend 1-pound weights to start.

2. Exhale, stretching to the right and keeping the weights an even distance apart. Don't allow your arms to collapse together. Pull your abdomen in and tighten your buttocks. Hold for a breath. Inhale and come back to center.

3. Exhale; repeat to the left.

4. Repeat 3 times.

# Gentle Yoga

## Gentle Yoga for Everyone

One beauty of yoga is that it can be enjoyed by everyone. Regardless of your size, shape, age, or fitness level, this gentle yet powerful discipline offers a completely balanced workout that will help you become leaner, stronger, and healthier. If you're very overweight or out of shape, or you're an absolute beginner, starting with a Gentle Yoga Workout will build your confidence and help you benefit from yoga without injury or strain. If you've recently had a baby, this is also the perfect workout for you. Gentle Yoga practice will teach you how to work within your fitness zone and respect your level of ability, strength, and flexibility.

Yoga is not the exclusive domain of young, ultra flexible, beautiful people, although the media often portray it that way. On the contrary, yoga's greatest benefits are for those who need the most help. People with full-sized bodies, heavy arms and thighs, or large stomachs may be intimidated by the challenge of apparently difficult, pretzel-like yoga poses. But with patience and perseverance, everyone can enrich their lives by practicing the Gentle Yoga routines in this chapter. They will safely and gradually allow you to increase your workout intensity, which will help you build your fitness level, regardless of where you start.

Gentle Yoga will tone and strengthen your legs, hips, buttocks, and abdomen and jump-start your metabolism to help you lose weight. Over time, yoga will help you shed unwanted pounds and, more important, help you discover what it means to be healthy and strong—not just thin. Yoga's path to peace of mind, body awareness, and self-acceptance will also encourage a healthy approach to food.

## Chair Yoga

Yoga can be modified for anyone who is carrying extra weight, or who has limited flexibility, tight joints, or other physical challenges. If you have difficulty lying or sitting on the floor, you can do Gentle

Yoga in a chair or on the edge of a bed. You can derive the benefits of many classic yoga poses in a chair or using a chair for support.

Proceed slowly, safely, and with awareness. Work the poses at your comfort level. Don't ever strain or force your body to the point of pain. Remember, the practice of yoga is the antithesis of the no-pain, no-gain approach to working out.

## Modify the Poses

Once you're comfortable with chair yoga and you begin to gain strength and flexibility, you'll want to progress to the next level by modifying your yoga poses with props such as a wall, bolster, blankets, blocks, pillows, and belts or straps. These props can help you compensate for physical limitations, such as difficulty reaching your arms above your head or sitting on the floor due to stiffness or expansive girth. The use of props will help prevent muscle, back, and knee strain due to weakness, lack of flexibility, or excess weight. For example, placing a folded blanket or a flat pillow beneath your sit bones (the lower points of the ischium) to elevate your hips will help you sit comfortably on the floor in Easy Pose (page 167). If you can't stretch forward, using a strap around the ball of your foot in Modified Head-to-Knee Pose (page 166) will help you extend your reach. A strap will also provide a safe stretch for tight hamstrings, as shown in Modified Reclining Big Toe Pose (page 165).

Standing postures and inverted ones can present a challenge for overweight people. Difficulty breathing and balancing in a Standing Forward Bend can be alleviated with the use of a block, as demonstrated in Modified Spread-Leg Forward Bend (page 158). Standing poses, such as Modified Tree Pose (page 159), develop balance and strength, and can be safely practiced with a chair or nearby wall if your balance feels wobbly. Headstands and shoulderstands can increase the risk of spinal injury and should be avoided, but the legs can be elevated safely against a wall so that you can derive the benefits of an inverted pose, as shown in Legs-up-the-Wall Pose (page 163).

As you progress, grow stronger, and improve with this Gentle Yoga program, you will naturally want to challenge yourself—and you should—with the routines in Chapters 3, 4, and 5. With steady practice (modifying the poses with props as needed) and a healthy, balanced diet, you will soon feel your body growing stronger. You'll notice excess pounds melting away and you'll feel calmer, more self-accepting, and more optimistic.

## After the Baby

You've just had a baby. Congratulations! Gentle Yoga is the best way to ease back into a regular exercise routine to regain and even improve your prepregnancy shape. Once you receive health clearance from your physician, you can begin the Yoga Basics and Gentle Yoga Workout outlined below. As you gain strength and muscle tone, you may want to switch to the routine in Chapter 4, "Yoga for Abdominals," to get your stomach muscles back into shape, or Chapter 3, "Yoga Power Workout," to lose weight. By combining a healthy, balanced diet with yoga, you will soon enjoy a new, improved postpregnancy physique.

## Yoga Basics and
## Gentle Yoga Workout Plan

Begin your first 2 weeks of yoga practice with the following Gentle Yoga poses and the Yoga Basics poses found in Chapter 2. Be aware that it may take you more than 2 weeks to do this routine comfortably, depending on your physical condition. If you feel comfortable and confident doing these poses, proceed to the Yoga Power Workouts found in Chapter 3. Otherwise, stay with Weeks 1 and 2 until you feel strong enough to continue.

## Week 1

**Workout Schedule:** Practice for 30 minutes, 3 or 4 times a week. Begin with Yoga Basics poses, proceed to Gentle Yoga poses, and then cool down with a few more Yoga Basics poses.

**Warm Up:**
Shoulder Press and Squeeze
Pelvic Tilt
Mountain Pose and Lifting the Sternum
Chest Expander

**Gentle Yoga:**
Seated Forward Hang
Seated Wheel Pose
Seated Side-to-Side
Seated Twist
Seated Triangle Pose
Seated Chest Expander

**Cool Down:**

Mula Bandha

Ujjayi Pranayama

Seated or Supported Relaxation Pose and Observation Meditation

## Week 2

**Workout Schedule:** Practice for 30 to 40 minutes, 4 times a week. Begin with Yoga Basics poses, proceed to Gentle Yoga poses, and then cool down with a few more Yoga Basics poses.

**Warm Up:**

Shoulder Press and Squeeze

Pelvic Tilt

Mountain Pose and Lifting the Sternum

Chest Expander

**Gentle Yoga:**

Modified Spread-Leg Forward Bend

Modified Tree Pose

Modified Warrior I

Modified Warrior III

Legs-up-the-Wall Pose
Modified Child's Pose
Modified Reclining Big Toe Pose

**Cool Down:**
Mula Bandha
Ujjayi Pranayama
Seated or Supported Relaxation Pose and Observation Meditation

## Gentle Yoga Asanas

## SEATED FORWARD HANG *(MODIFIED UTTANASANA)*

**What It Does:** It stretches the back, tones the abdominals, calms the nerves, and quiets the mind. As you build strength, practice Modified Spread-Leg Forward Bend (page 158).

**How to Do It:**

1. Sit straight in a chair with your legs together and your feet flat on the floor.

2. Inhale. Exhale, rounding your shoulders and relaxing your spine forward, one vertebra at a time. Lower your forehead to your knees, resting your chest on your thighs as your arms hang down by your legs. Feel your back and shoulder muscles stretch as you relax in the position for 3 breaths.

3. Place your hands on your knees and slowly roll up, one vertebra at a time, raising your head last, to upright seated position. Repeat.

## SEATED WHEEL POSE
## (MODIFIED CHAKRASANA)

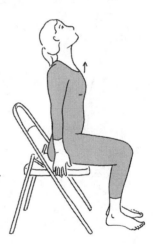

**What It Does:** It increases spinal flexibility, improves breathing, tones the internal organs, and improves posture.

**How to Do It:**

1. Sit straight at the edge of your chair with feet flat on the floor, hands resting on the armrests or lightly on the seat of the chair.

2. Inhale and arch, lifting your breastbone. Lift your chin and gaze upward. Do not crunch your neck as you bring your chin up;

bring your head back only as far as you can support it. Hold for 3 breaths.

3. Release to a relaxed seated position.

## SEATED SIDE-TO-SIDE (MODIFIED NITAMBASANA)

**What It Does:** It releases tension and fatigue and tones the upper body. This is a simpler version of Standing Side-to-Side (page 61) and Side Bend with Weights (page 142).

**How to Do It:**

1. Sit straight in a chair with your feet flat on the floor. Inhale, raising your arms up beside your ears, your palms facing each other. Stretch your torso and rib cage upward.

2. Exhale, stretching to the right. Pull your abdomen in. Look under your left arm. Come to center. Repeat left.

3. Lower your arms and come to a relaxed seated position.

# SEATED TWIST
## (MODIFIED BHARADVAJASANA)

**What It Does:** It increases spine and neck flexibility; releases tension and fatigue from back muscles.

**How to Do It:**

1. Sit straight in a chair with legs together and feet flat on the floor. Inhale, lengthen your spine, and place your left hand on your right knee and your right hand on the back of the chair.

2. Exhale and gently twist your body right—turn your belly, then your chest, then your shoulders, then your head, directing your gaze over your right shoulder. Keep your shoulder blades down and in. Hold for 3 breaths.

3. Slowly return to center, beginning with the belly, then the chest, shoulder, head, and eyes.

4. Repeat the twist to the left.

# SEATED TRIANGLE POSE
## (MODIFIED TRIKONASANA)

**What It Does:** It stretches and tones the muscles of the back, arms, and ribs. This is a simpler version of Triangle (page 87).

**How to Do It:**

1. Sit straight in a chair with legs together and feet flat on the floor. Inhale and raise your arms to a T position.

2. Exhale, twist, and bring your right hand down to your left foot on floor. Raise your left hand toward the ceiling and look up. Hold for 3 breaths.

3. Return to an upright sitting position.

4. Repeat to the left.

# SEATED CHEST EXPANDER

**What It Does:** It opens the chest, relieves tension and tightness in the back, neck, and shoulders, and improves posture. This is a simpler version of Chest Expander (page 29).

**How to Do It:**

1. Sit at the edge of your chair with legs together, feet flat on the floor, and spine straight. Clasp your hands behind your back and gently squeeze your shoulder blades together.

2. Inhale, straightening your elbows, expanding your chest, and lifting your arms and chin. Exhale, folding forward from the hips and bringing your chest to your thighs, hands clasped above your head.

3. Inhale, slowly rise to upright seated position, and rest your clasped hands on the back of the chair. If your hands can't reach the top of the chair back, then clasp the sides of the chair back. Exhale, gently squeezing your shoulder blades together, lifting your chin, and dropping your head back. Hold for 2 breaths.

4. Exhale, release your hands, and return to a relaxed seated position. Repeat.

# MODIFIED SPREAD-LEG FORWARD BEND
## (MODIFIED PRASARITA PADA UTTANASANA)

**What It Does:** Performed with a block, this will help release and stretch tight hips and hamstrings and prevent lower-back strain. Use an appropriately sized block or similar prop that suits your flexibility needs or limitations. As you grow stronger and more flexible, you may wish to replace the block with a book, until you can comfortably reach the floor with your hands.

**How to Do It:**

1. Place the block about a foot in front of you between your wide-spread legs (your feet should be 3 to 4 feet apart).

2. Inhale, then exhale, folding forward from the hips and placing your hands on the block. Pull your abdomen in.

3. Hang comfortably for 6 to 8 breaths.

4. Come to standing, pulling your abdominals in.

# MODIFIED TREE POSE *(MODIFIED VRKSASANA)*

**What It Does:** It improves balance, strengthens legs, and increases the flexibility of the hips and groin. A belt or strap will help keep your foot from slipping and maintain your hip's open position. As you grow stronger, more confident and balanced, remove the strap and practice the pose alongside a wall or chair for additional support.

**How to Do It:**

1. Wrap a belt or strap around your bent right ankle and thigh, holding the ends with your right hand. Place the sole of your right foot at the top of your left inner thigh, bringing the foot as high up the leg as possible. With your left hand, hold on to a chair or wall. Press your right knee back, trying to bring it in line with your right hip.

2. Gaze at a spot on the floor, but keep your eyes soft. Breathe gently.

3. If you have your balance, raise your left hand a few inches

off the chair. Hold the pose for 3 or 4 breaths. If you sway or wobble, don't give up. Simply lean on the chair or wall to regain your balance before trying again.

4. Bring your right foot down slowly, letting the belt slip off your leg (control the motion). Stand steady with both feet firmly grounded.

5. Repeat on the other side.

## MODIFIED WARRIOR I
### (MODIFIED VIRABHADRASANA I)

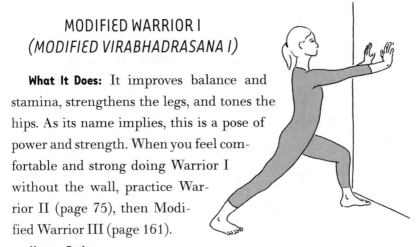

**What It Does:** It improves balance and stamina, strengthens the legs, and tones the hips. As its name implies, this is a pose of power and strength. When you feel comfortable and strong doing Warrior I without the wall, practice Warrior II (page 75), then Modified Warrior III (page 161).

**How to Do It:**

1. Place your hands on the wall shoulder-width apart and a little above shoulder height. Stand with your feet 3 to 4 feet apart, the left

foot facing forward with toes touching the wall and the right foot turned out.

2. Bend your left leg until it is close to a right angle. Right leg is straight. Square your hips to face the wall. Press your shoulder blades down as you push against the wall with your hands.

3. Inhale and straighten your left leg, keeping your hands against the wall. Exhale and bend the left leg. Repeat 2 times.

4. Repeat the pose on the other side. As you grow stronger and more confident, and you no longer need to lean against the wall for support, raise both arms over your head with your palms facing each other.

## MODIFIED WARRIOR III
## *(MODIFIED VIRABHADRASANA III)*

**What It Does:** It improves balance and stamina, strengthens the legs, and tones the hips and abdominals.

**How to Do It:**

1. Stand with legs close together in Mountain Pose (page 84), about 2 feet from the wall. Lean forward and place both hands on the wall shoulder-width apart and above shoulder height. Press

your shoulder blades down as you push against the wall with your hands.

2. Exhale and slowly lift the left leg back. Straighten your left leg by actively pushing out through the heel. Keep the right leg straight and rooted to the ground. Gaze at a spot on the floor, but keep your eyes soft. Breathe gently.

3. Return to Mountain Pose. Repeat Warrior III on the other side.

As you grow stronger and more confident and no longer need the wall to balance, give yourself enough room to extend both arms in front of you without touching the wall. Gaze at your outstretched hands.

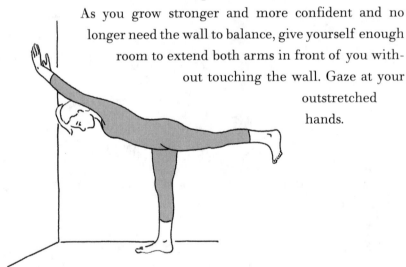

# LEGS-UP-THE-WALL POSE *(MODIFIED VIPARITA KARANI)*

**What It Does:** This is a safe and simple way to get all the benefits of an inversion posture. It improves circulation to the upper body and head and calms the mind. When you grow stronger and more flexible and confident, practice Half Shoulderstand (page 126).

**How to Do It:**

1. Sit on the floor beside the wall, with one shoulder as close to the wall as possible. Knees are bent.

2. Swing around and bring both legs up against the wall as you lie back on the floor. Extend your legs straight up the wall with your arms at your sides, keeping your buttocks against the wall. Breathing comfortably, stay in this position for 1 minute.

3. If your hamstring muscles are stiff and tight, bend your knees a bit. If your lower back, shoulders, and neck are uncomfortable, place a folded blanket or towel beneath them.

4. Come out of the pose by bending your knees, turning to one side, and slowly sitting up. Follow Legs-up-the-Wall with Modified Child's Pose, which follows.

## MODIFIED CHILD'S POSE *(MODIFIED SALAMBA BALASANA)*

**What It Does:** Try this restful pose after backbends and inversion poses. Modified Child's Pose provides deep relaxation and relieves back tension and fatigue.

### How to Do It:

1. Kneel in front of a bolster or folded blankets. Knees are spread wide, with big toes touching. Put the bolster between your thighs, drawn up to the groin. If sitting on your ankles is uncomfortable, place a pillow under your ankles.

2. Inhale, then exhale slowly and bend forward, lowering your torso to rest on the bolster. Relax your arms around the support. Turn your face to one side. Relax deeply. Breathe comfortably.

3. Rest for as long as you wish.

# MODIFIED RECLINING BIG TOE POSE
## (MODIFIED SUPTA PADANGUSTHASANA)

**What It Does:** It increases the flexibility and strength of the hamstrings and legs and provides preparation for all poses.

**How to Do It:**

1. Lie on your back with both knees bent, the soles of your feet flat on the floor. Wrap a belt or strap around the ball of your right foot.

2. Inhale and straighten your right leg toward the ceiling. Exhale, tilting the pelvis under. If you're unable to fully straighten the right leg, keep it bent, so that your sit bones drop toward the ground.

3. Inhale and bend the right leg. Exhale and straighten the right leg again, to the point where you are stretching comfortably but any further stretching would cause discomfort. Draw the right leg closer to your face, applying gentle leverage with the belt. Work up to holding for 2 or 3 breaths.

4. As you grow more flexible, keep your right leg straight and ac-

tively straighten your left leg, pressing the back of the leg into the floor. Actively push out through the heels of both feet. Return the right leg to the floor.

5. Repeat on the other side. Once you've established this basic pose, practice without the belt, placing both hands around your thigh, calf, or ankle.

## MODIFIED HEAD-TO-KNEE POSE (MODIFIED JANU SIRSASANA)

**What It Does:** It increases the flexibility and strength of the spine, hips, and legs and tones the abdomen and abdominal organs. As you grow more flexible, remove the belt and the blanket and gradually work up to Seated Forward Bend (page 107).

**How to Do It:**

1. Sit on the floor, with a folded blanket under your hips and your legs extended out in front of you. Bend your right leg and rest the sole of your right foot on your left groin. Wrap a belt or strap around the ball of your left foot.

2. Inhale and lengthen your torso, pulling up from the waist, letting your sternum rise. Press your shoulder blades down.

3. Exhale and fold forward, leading with the sternum and rotating to the left in order to center your torso over your straight left leg. Allow your pelvis to rotate forward with the spine in a straight line. Don't curve the upper back as you reach forward. If you feel pain or discomfort in your back or leg, bend your left leg as much as necessary to alleviate it. Never force yourself.

4. Inhale and elongate your spine, lengthening your torso forward. Exhale and stretch to your edge, the point beyond which you would feel discomfort. Work up to holding for 2 or 3 breaths.

5. Inhale and come up slowly. Repeat on the other side.

## EASY POSE *(SUKHASANA)*

**What It Does:** This restful pose increases flexibility in the hips, legs, and ankles. It is used for meditation and the cultivation of calmness.

**How to Do It:**

1. Sit on the floor on the edge of a folded blanket to support your hips. Cross your legs. Sit with your spine straight. Your knees should be lower than the top of your pelvis. If your back is rounded, or your

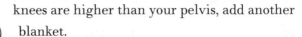

knees are higher than your pelvis, add another blanket.

2. Place your hands on your knees, palms turned up. Close your eyes and bring your attention to your breath. Practice Observation Meditation (page 32).

3. As your flexibility increases, forego the blanket and sit directly on the floor, centered on your sit bones.

## SUPPORTED RELAXATION POSE
### (SUPPORTED SAVASANA)

**What It Does:** It enhances the effectiveness of the poses, calms the mind and nervous system, and helps relieve insomnia. End your yoga toning practice with this pose or the Seated Relaxation Pose that follows.

**How to Do It:**

1. Lie on your back on a mat on the floor with a folded blanket under your head and neck. You may want to put an additional folded blanket or two under your back.

2. Place your feet a comfortable distance apart. Hands are at sides, palms turned upward. Move your shoulders down and away from your ears, and tuck the shoulder blades in toward your spine. If your back feels uncomfortable with your legs straight, bend your knees as much as you need to, to alleviate pain or discomfort. You may feel more comfortable with a folded blanket or pillow underneath your knees.

3. Inhale; exhale, contracting the buttock muscles and pressing the curve out of your lower back. Release and relax completely.

4. Relax each part of your body. Begin by focusing your attention on your feet and toes. Inhale and suggest to your feet and toes that they relax. Exhale and feel your feet and toes relaxing. Repeat this relaxation procedure with each individual body part.

5. Practice Observation Meditation (page 32).

6. Relax all efforts and rest in the stillness for as long as you wish.

# SEATED RELAXATION POSE *(MODIFIED SAVASANA)*

**What It Does:** Always end your yoga practice with a Relaxation Pose. This will enhance the effectiveness of all that's come before. It will calm your mind and nervous system and help to relieve insomnia. This is a seated version of Supported Relaxation Pose (page 168), which is done lying down.

**How to Do It:**

1. Sit straight in a chair with feet flat on the floor and shoes off, keeping your back straight and your neck and head aligned with your spinal column. Close your eyes and rest your hands in your lap. Breathe through your nose, peaceful and relaxed.

2. Relax each part of your body. Begin by focusing your attention on your feet and toes. Inhale and suggest to your feet and toes that they relax. Exhale and feel your feet and toes relaxing. Repeat this relaxation procedure with each individual body part.

3. Practice Observation Meditation (page 32).

4. Relax all efforts and rest in the stillness for as long as you wish.

# Yoga Food

## Battle of the Bulge

From Atkins to the Zone, Blood Type to Sugar Busters, there are more fad diets out there than there are calories in a Big Mac. Every day, millions of Americans are trying to lose weight, and most of the weight they lose, they will regain quickly. When you go off these fad diets, as you inevitably do, how can you maintain the weight loss you've achieved? More important, with all the hype and conflicting theories, how do you choose the best nutritional plan for your body and your needs?

Simple answers can be found in Eastern and Western holistic traditions; they include practicing yoga and incorporating practices of Ayurveda and the world's healthiest cuisines. Since fad diets are by nature unsuccessful in the long term, why not try weight management from a holistic perspective that encompasses the mind, body, and spirit? By balancing food intake, exercise, and meditation, you'll shed pounds while enriching your mind. You'll achieve a lifetime of weight loss success as you enjoy delicious, healthful eating and glowing good health.

## The World's Healthiest Diets

The world's healthiest diets, including vegetarian, Mediterranean, and Asian diets, share several important components that contribute to successful weight loss and maintenance.

### PORTION CONTROL

The most healthful way to reach and maintain your ideal weight is to eat smaller portions of a variety of healthful foods. By including more whole grains, beans, vegetables, herbs, and flavorful spices and reducing your meat consumption, you can enjoy your meals and never feel deprived.

To get an idea of correct portions, keep in mind that the recommended 4-ounce serving of chicken and 3-ounce serving of fish are each about the size of a deck of cards, $^1/_2$ cup of high-fiber whole grains is about the size of a golf ball, and 1 cup of vegetables is about the size of a tennis ball.

## MINDFUL EATING

Ayurveda, yoga philosophy, and the Asian diet endorse a mindful eating practice for optimal health. Practice a state of awareness while you eat; savor the appearance, smell, and taste of your food, so that you can be truly satisfied by your meal. Eat slowly, in a calm, quiet environment without the accompaniment of a blaring television or your computer. Such distractions often make people unaware that they're eating too quickly or overeating.

Ayurveda calls the ultimate and essential nature of things *rasa*, or the "juice" of an object. Explore the rasa of your food through your five senses. See, smell, touch, taste, and observe any sounds as you eat the food. Does the food bring you any satisfaction after you eat it? You may notice the preservatives and artificial flavors of your favorite junk foods, and realize they weren't as delicious as you previously thought. A piece of fresh, ripe fruit may ultimately hold more appeal to your awakened senses.

## EATING LESS MEAT

In the world's healthiest diets, an ounce or two of poultry per person is used a few times a week and red meat is included, as a condiment, only a few times a month. This meat restriction arose from a scarcity of meat in these global cultures, but it had the result of dramatically lowering the saturated fat in their diets. Only small amounts of meat are used to flavor vegetable-, legume-, and grain-based dishes. Fish is eaten in moderate portions weekly.

## INCLUDING FAT-FREE HERBS AND SPICES

Instead of depending on butter and other high-fat dressings to flavor foods, experiment with fat-free condiments, herbs, and spices. Try international condiments such as soy sauce, fish sauce, miso (Japanese fermented bean paste), rice wine vinegar, balsamic vinegar, and black bean sauce. Experiment with a variety of fresh herbs and spices, such as ginger, garlic, lemongrass, basil, oregano, thyme, rosemary, hot peppers, cinnamon, turmeric, and Asian five-spice powder (a combination of Szechwan peppercorns, fennel seed, star anise, cinnamon, and cloves).

# USING DAIRY PRODUCTS JUDICIOUSLY

Milk and other dairy products have been an integral part of global cuisine for millennia. Milk and the sacred cow have an important status in Indian and yogic culture; and milk, yogurt, and ghee (clarified butter) are an essential part of a sattvic diet. Yogis also believe that eating these types of dairy products strengthens deep meditation. Studies have shown that the amino acid tryptophan, found in milk (among the protein foods), does encourage a feeling of calm and relaxation. Milk has also been found to be an excellent source of calcium (an 8-ounce serving of 2-percent-fat milk has 135 mg of calcium) and other vitamins and minerals. As a source of protein, low-fat milk can be a healthy alternative to meat.

However, there has been much nutritional debate about the quality of our milk supply. Nonorganic cow's milk and other dairy products are laced with antibiotics, synthetic growth hormones, and pesticides, all of which could have dangerous health effects. In addition, the saturated fat and cholesterol found in whole milk and full-fat dairy products increase your risk of heart disease. The best alternative is to choose nonfat and low-fat organic dairy products. The world's healthiest diets recommend that dairy foods be eaten in small quantities, preferably about 1 cup daily. Many experts believe these recommendations and restrictions are crucial for controlling obesity and maintaining ideal weight.

You may also want to try tasty dairy alternatives, such as soy-, rice-, and grain-based beverages and foods. Other substitutions to enjoy are goat milk products, such as goat cheese and nonfat goat yogurt.

## Lose Weight with Ayurveda

Your weight loss program doesn't have to be a grim regimen of cutting calories and exercising an hour a day to lose that pound a week. Instead, try embracing Ayurveda, the ancient Indian healing system for the mind, body, and spirit. Ayurveda, or "the science of life," offers a holistic program to achieve perfect health and ideal weight by balancing all the elements of your life. Ayurveda, a five-thousand-year-old healing system, views excess weight, or obesity, as a sign of a body out of balance. The goal of ayurvedic medicine is to achieve perfect health and balance of the mind, body, and spirit through proper nutrition, exercise, and meditation. Restoring ayurvedic balance is the means to losing excess weight. The first step is to correct any digestive problems. Then Ayurveda guides you to the appropriate selection of food, drink, and herbs to improve metabolic efficiency.

Ayurveda is based on the theory of the three *doshas*, or mind-body types, which have their own set of physical, mental, and emotional characteristics. The three doshas are *vata* (air), *pitta* (fire), and *kapha* (earth). All people and things possess elements of each dosha, but one or more of the doshas may predominate in your body and behavior. For example, you may be a vata-pitta, a pitta-kapha, or a vata-kapha. Your unique combination of doshas is your constitution type, or *prakruti*, which establishes your physical, mental, and emotional makeup. One way to achieve balance and ideal weight through Ayurveda is to identify your dosha, then make appropriate adjustments in diet, yoga practice, and lifestyle.

## What's Your Dosha?

To determine which dosha is most dominant in your body, make a check mark over the individual characteristics (listed below) that describe you. The category with the most check marks will indicate your dosha. If you have almost the same number of checks marks in two or more categories, your body type is a mixture of two or three doshas. This list of characteristics will give only a rough indication of your dosha. Accurately determining your dosha body type is best left to an ayurvedic physician.

## BODY TYPE: VATA

**Physical Characteristics:** Thin, light-boned, angular build; slow to gain weight; dry skin and hair; eats and sleeps erratically; chilly hands and feet; low ratio of muscle to fat; fat accumulates below the navel (prone to potbelly on a lean frame).

**Mental Characteristics:** Quick mind; restlessness; creates and learns quickly; forgets easily; enthusiastic; imaginative; vivacious.

**Emotional Characteristics:** Prone to anxiety, worry, mood swings, and nervous disorders.

**Diet:** Benefits from grounding foods, such as grains and oils.

## BODY TYPE: PITTA

**Physical Characteristics:** Medium-sized, athletic build; well proportioned; blond, red, or prematurely gray hair; fair or freckled complexion; warm, ruddy, perspiring skin; good stamina; voracious appetite and tendency to overeat; tends to be warm or hot; sleeps well; eats meals quickly; likely to develop ulcers; gains and loses weight easily; apple shape when overweight.

**Mental Characteristics:** Confident, passionate, articulate, courageous, intelligent, ambitious.

**Emotional Characteristics:** Demanding, irritable, impatient, short-tempered.

**Diet:** Benefits from cooling foods, such as salads and sweet fruits.

## BODY TYPE: KAPHA

**Physical Characteristics:** Large, heavy build; wide shoulders; voluptuous or barrel-chested; gains weight easily and has trouble losing it; thick, moist skin and lustrous hair; difficulty with digestion; prone to respiratory illness; excellent stamina; needs more sleep than vata or pitta; eats slowly; pear shape when overweight.

**Mental Characteristics:** Forgiving, affectionate, relaxed, slow and graceful, slow to anger, calm, tolerant, reliable.

**Emotional Characteristics:** Lethargy, procrastination, depression.

**Diet:** Benefits from heating and invigorating foods, such as cayenne and other hot spices.

## The Three Nutritional Gunas

The ayurvedic principle of the three *gunas*—*sattva, rajas,* and *tamas*—describes the basic constituents found in nature. These three forces exist in limitless combinations in the universe.

- *Sattva* is the principle of purity and the balancing force that harmonizes the positive and negative.
- *Rajas* is the principle of activity and the positive force that initiates change.
- *Tamas* is the principle of inactivity and the negative force that sustains previous activity.

The ayurvedic and yogic view of nutrition is traditionally divided into these three gunas.

Sattvic foods are pure and life-giving, and they promote health, vitality, strength, serenity, and relaxation. These foods are organically grown, additive- and preservative-free, and unprocessed. They include fresh fruits and juices, vegetables and herbs, whole grain cereals, nuts and seeds, peas, beans, lentils, dairy, and natural sweeteners such as honey and molasses.

Rajasic foods are overstimulating and promote excess energy, agitation, discontent, and disease. These foods are spicy, sour, salty, pungent, bitter, overly hot, and dry. They include all meat, all fish, eggs, hot peppers, most spices, and coffee, tea, and other caffeine beverages.

Tamasic foods are stale, old, spoiled, impure, rotten, overly processed, additive- and preservative-filled, and addictive. These foods dull the mind and promote overeating, addiction, inactivity, laziness, and lethargy. They include tobacco, drugs, shriveled fruits and vegetables, mushrooms, and processed, packaged, preserved, or deep-fried foods.

Yogis eat mainly organic sattvic foods, which promote the life force of the body. They limit their use of rajasic and tamasic foods, or eliminate them whenever possible. Not all yogis are vegetarians, but those who do eat meat do so in moderation. Yogis believe that meat has a low vibration or life force and its inherent toxins will reduce the vitality of the person eating it. They believe that fresh, organic fruits and vegetables possess the highest vibration and life force of all foods.

Yogis also believe that how and when you eat is as important as what you eat. To extract all nutrients from foods and eliminate toxins, they eat slowly and with awareness, and they don't combine eating with other activities, such as watching television. They observe mitahara, or moderation in all things, and they don't eat too much or too often. Yogis eat only when they're truly hungry, not when bored or upset, and limit the meal to fit their true appetite. They eat their most substantial meal at noon, when the digestive fires are strongest.

## Kapha Reducing Diet

Being overweight commonly indicates an out-of-balance kapha, but can also result from a pitta or vata imbalance. Individuals with a dominant kapha dosha tend to gain weight easily and have trouble losing weight. In many cases, they are overweight because their metabolisms (digestive fire, or *agni*) are sluggish. An ayurvedic weight loss program includes yoga practice, observing the principles of the three gunas and mitahara, and reducing kapha-aggravating foods in the diet, including heavy, sweet, sour, salty, oily, and greasy foods. Pungent, warming spices are part of the kapha diet because they light the fires of digestion.

The following are the essential components of a kapha reducing diet.

1. Eat leafy green vegetables, such as spinach, beet greens, dandelion greens, and lettuce; radishes; sprouts; and fresh fruits such as apples, pears, cherries, and berries.

2. Avoid all dairy products except skim or low-fat milk.

3. Limit or eliminate red meat. Eat skinless white turkey or chicken breast meat instead.

4. Eat whole grains such as corn, barley, and basmati rice, and beans and legumes such as garbanzos and red lentils.

5. Don't eat wheat; nuts; sweet, sour, salty, oily, or greasy foods; or prepared or refined foods.

6. Eliminate sweet, juicy fruits such as pineapple, watermelon, and papaya.

7. Drink warm beverages such as herbal teas or warm water sweetened with honey and lemon. Avoid cold beverages, including alcoholic drinks and sugary sodas.

8. Avoid foods made with refined sugar. Use honey as a sweetener instead.

9. Include warming, pungent spices, such as ginger, black pepper, cayenne, turmeric, cumin, coriander, fennel, and cinnamon, in your cooking.

10. Exercise regularly according to your dosha (see "Ayurveda Asanas," below).

## Ayurveda Asanas

An ayurvedic weight loss program features regular exercise, including yoga practice, tailored to your dosha. Include asanas that balance your constitution, or *prakruti*. Individuals of all doshas will benefit from practicing Sun Salutation (see Chapter 3, "Yoga Power Workout") and Savasana Relaxation (pages 168 and 170).

People of a *vata* constitution or imbalance benefit from light-to-moderate exercise, including walking, hiking, and cycling. Most yoga poses are calming, balancing, and grounding, and counter vata's agitated nature. However, vata asanas should be performed slowly and with awareness. For example, Sun Salutation vinyasas should be performed at a slow and thoughtful pace. Other asanas that are beneficial for vatas include Standing Forward Bend, Seated Forward Bend, Child's Pose, Easy Pose, and Bow Pose.

People of a *pitta* constitution or imbalance benefit from moderate exercise, including jogging, swimming, and cycling. Pitta individuals also benefit from calming, quieting yoga poses to counter their aggressive tendencies. They should perform Sun Salutation vinyasas at a moderate pace and with minimal repetitions. Other asanas that are beneficial for pittas include Cobra and Bow Pose.

People of a *kapha* constitution or imbalance benefit from intense cardiovascular exercise, including running, aerobics, and in-line skating. Kapha individuals benefit from daily exercise to counter their tendency toward lethargy and obesity. They should perform Sun Salutation vinyasas at an intense pace and with many repetitions. Other asanas that are beneficial for kaphas include Bridge Pose, abdominal poses (see Chapter 4), and Fish Pose.

## Fasting and Panchakarma

A yoga lifestyle is often identified with fasting practices. Many yoga and Ayurveda practitioners believe that fasting detoxifies the digestive system and aids in weight management while promoting healing and reversing aging. Fasting is also embraced as a way to practice self-discipline, deepen meditation and spirituality, and increase alertness and concentration. Studies have shown that fasting helps alleviate migraines, rheumatoid arthritis, and skin diseases. It may also help in the treatment of obesity, colon disorders, allergies, and respiratory illnesses. However, no substantial studies support fasting's detoxification claims.

Some experts believe that fasting depletes the body of essential nutrients and that it is not a particularly effective weight loss aid. It is believed that most of the weight lost during fasting is from water, and that this weight will return when the fast is over. Besides hunger pains, negative effects of fasting include low energy, weakness, headaches, and nausea. Fasting may be unsafe and is not recommended for pregnant or lactating women, diabetics, hypoglycemics, or individuals with eating disorders, ulcers, and other health conditions.

There are several types of fasting. A complete fast, in which you drink only water, is not recommended unless it will be medically supervised. A modified fast allows fruit or vegetable juices, herbal teas, and sometimes small portions of whole grains. It should be limited to no more than a few days and carried out under the supervision of a medical professional. A 1-day partial fast is the type most often recommended, as it is unlikely to cause any harm and is well tolerated by most healthy people.

In Ayurveda, the detoxification program of *panchakarma* includes a partial fast and a series of treatments that include massage using organic sesame oil, aromatherapy, herbal steam baths and herbal pastes to detoxify the body. The same foods are eaten for several days, usually a simple diet of mung lentils and rice. A panchakarma program is done under the supervision of an ayurvedic physician. Such programs are offered in ayurvedic group settings and yoga centers.

## Controlling Cravings with Ayurveda

Do you fantasize about devouring a bag of potato chips? Does your heart desire a pint of your favorite ice cream? Do you ever feel like your food cravings control you? Don't worry, it just means you're human. We all have cravings from time to time, and for some of us, fighting cravings is a daily struggle. However, these cravings can have detrimental effects if they result in weight gain and poor nutrition.

Cravings for refined carbohydrates such as pastries and chocolates are common. One of the most frequent causes of carb cravings is low blood sugar. This is usually caused by a diet that is high in refined carbohydrates. When we eat too many refined carbs—pastries, white bread, and sweets—our blood sugar rises quickly. The pancreas responds to this high blood sugar by oversecreting insulin, which may cause blood-sugar levels to drop precipitously, bringing on hypoglycemia. When blood-sugar levels and energy drop, the urge to eat more processed carbs or sweets can be very powerful.

Stress may contribute to cravings. When stressed, the body attempts to boost the brain's production of serotonin, a neurotransmitter that produces feelings of calm and well-being. This produces a craving for carbohydrates, raw ingredients the body needs to manufacture serotonin.

People may also crave protein-rich foods when under pressure: such foods have been associated with increased alertness, concentration, and performance. Women can crave chocolate and sweets during the 7 to 10 days before their periods; a premenstrual drop in serotonin may create an increase in appetite, and especially a craving for carbs.

Cooler weather can also stimulate appetite. Many people find themselves eating more and exercising less then. That can be a problem if you're struggling to maintain a healthy weight.

According to Ayurveda, food cravings represent an imbalance. Kapha constitutions or imbalances are attracted to foods like their own nature, heavy and sweet. To help control these cravings, Ayurveda recommends including six tastes at every meal: sweet, sour, salty, bitter, pungent, and astringent; these can be inherent in your food choices or added with ayurvedic spice mixtures.

Some sweet foods to include in your diet are honey and kapha-diet fruits such as apples, pears, cherries, and berries. The recommended sour foods include nonfat yogurt and vinegar. The salty foods include sea vegetables. The bitter foods include turmeric and green leafy vegetables such as spinach and dandelion greens. The pungent foods include ginger, black pepper, and cayenne. The astringent foods include beans and lentils.

Other ways to control cravings include exercise. With regular workouts, your mood swings and cravings can disappear. Exercise also reduces stress and increases your energy. Studies have found that even a brisk walk before a meal reduces appetite and the urge to snack.

It's helpful to eat a varied diet that's low in sugar and has a balanced distribution of protein from low-fat animal or vegetable sources and low-glycemic-index carbs—ones that don't raise blood sugar levels as quickly, such as whole grains, legumes, and vegetables. You should also eat healthy fats such as olive and flaxseed oils. These foods will keep blood sugar at an even keel and help prevent extreme blood-sugar fluctuations and cravings.

In addition, consider keeping a food-craving diary for a few months. Note everything you eat and drink and the times you crave sweets. By keeping a record you may begin to see dietary patterns that provide the key to ending your cravings. For instance, you may have a daily craving for a candy bar around 4 p.m. Try to anticipate this urge and eat a healthful, low-fat, low-calorie snack at 3:30. This will negate your urge for the candy bar.

A good strategy for preventing food cravings is to eat healthy snacks every few hours throughout the day to keep blood-sugar levels steady. These healthy snacks can include fresh veggies, low-fat yogurt, or an apple. When you'll be away from home, take along protein-rich snacks such as nutrient-balanced energy bars, trail mix, nuts, seeds, or low-fat cheese strips for when your energy level drops.

# Index

# About the Author

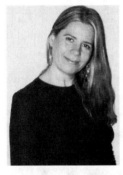

ELAINE GAVALAS received her master's degree from Columbia University, New York. She's an exercise physiologist, health expert, and weight management specialist who works with groups and individuals of all sizes, shapes, and ages to help them reach and maintain their ideal weight, wellness, and fitness goals. She utilizes yoga and fitness techniques that integrate the body, mind, and spirit.

Her yoga minibook series includes *The Yoga Minibook for Weight Loss, The Yoga Minibook for Stress Relief, The Yoga Minibook for Longevity,* and *The Yoga Minibook for Energy and Strength.* Gavalas is also the author of numerous yoga, fitness, and diet articles and books, including *Secrets of Fat-Free Greek Cooking* (1998).

If you or your company would like to contact Elaine or want more information about her books, videotapes, or group and individual services, visit her website at www.yogaminibooks.com or e-mail her at AskElaineG@aol.com.

# Exercise your body, soul, and mind with the entire series of Yoga Minibooks

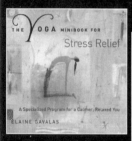

**The Yoga Minibook for Stress Relief**

0-7432-2701-8 · $10.00

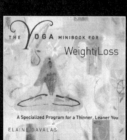

**The Yoga Minibook for Weight Loss**

0-7432-2698-4 · $10.00

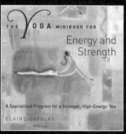

**The Yoga Minibook for Energy and Strength**

0-7432-2700-X · $10.00

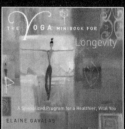

**The Yoga Minibook for Longevity**

0-7432-2699-2 · $10.00

**FIRESIDE**
A Division of Simon & Schuster
A VIACOM COMPANY